End Pain

&

Feel Great Again!

Other Resources by the Author
available at: *store.duncantooley.com*

Healthy & Feeling Great
- *Medical Benefits of Hypnosis* – free report
- *Feel Great* hypnotic pain relief & wellness meditation
- *60-second Pain Relief* process
- *Pain Gone* word search puzzle
- *More Fun Exercise* meditation
- *Anti-Anxious* word search puzzles
- *Self-Hypnosis to Accelerate Healing* multimedia meditation
- *Knockout Stress* multimedia experience
- *Restful Sleep Expels Insomnia* meditation

Positivity-Creativity-Art-Fun
- *Tooley's Law* (of Attraction) – free audio
- *Principles of Tooley's Law* (of Attraction)
- *Fun Creative Art* word search puzzle
- *Creative Mandala Experience* multimedia meditation
- *Positive Aspects* word search puzzles
- *Ace My Exam or Final Grade* meditation experience
- *Increase Anything* meditation experience

Nutrition & Weight
- *Think Myself SLIM® Weight Loss System* – free sample
- *Turn Your Fat Burner UP* hypnotic meditation
- *Healthy Eating* word search puzzle
- *End My French Fry Craving* multimedia
- *Turn OFF ANY Craving* multimedia meditation
- *Tap Away Overeating* acupressure process

Resource information at *store.duncantooley.com*

Email Contact: *duncan@duncantooley.com*
Or call **310-832-0830**
Also see artworks by the author at: *www.TooleyArtStudio.com,*
and more pain-related information at: *www.painhypnotist.com*

Is this book my *PAIN RELIEF ANSWER?*

"It's almost like a magic spell. I have no pain. I have my old life back, able to do everything I want pain-free." -- Rebecca Harris"

It was amazing! Duncan's process stopped my serious pain from six surgeries and a fused ankle." -- Shelley Fine

"Ten years of chronic pain instantly decreased dramatically. I stopped taking six Codeine pills a day." -- Jane Smolens

"Duncan Tooley taught me how to turn off the pain, calm the itching, and make my red skin bumps disappear... I had no idea that I could easily have control over my pain." -- Dina Wiley

"Duncan Tooley shows that you can become pain free. You don't have you don't have to struggle with pain for years, or accept being in pain as a normal way of life."-- Dr. Leyla Ali, Pharmacist and Author of *Off Balance, The American Way of Health, A Pharmacist's Perspective on Why Drugs Don't Work.*

"If you want relief, this book is a must read."-- Shelley Stockwell Nicholas, PhD, President, International Hypnosis Federation.

"Duncan Tooley generously shares how to communicate with pain, and then use your will, intention, and mind to repair and restore. Almost too simple and effective to be believed! It just works!"-- Dr. Aviva Boxer, OMD, (DrAvivaBoxer.com) "Restoring radiant vitality, resilience and stamina without an expiration date."

"When I had my back incident, I could not get up off the floor until I used Tooley's 60-second Turn Down technique"-- Glen Michael

My Powerful Mind

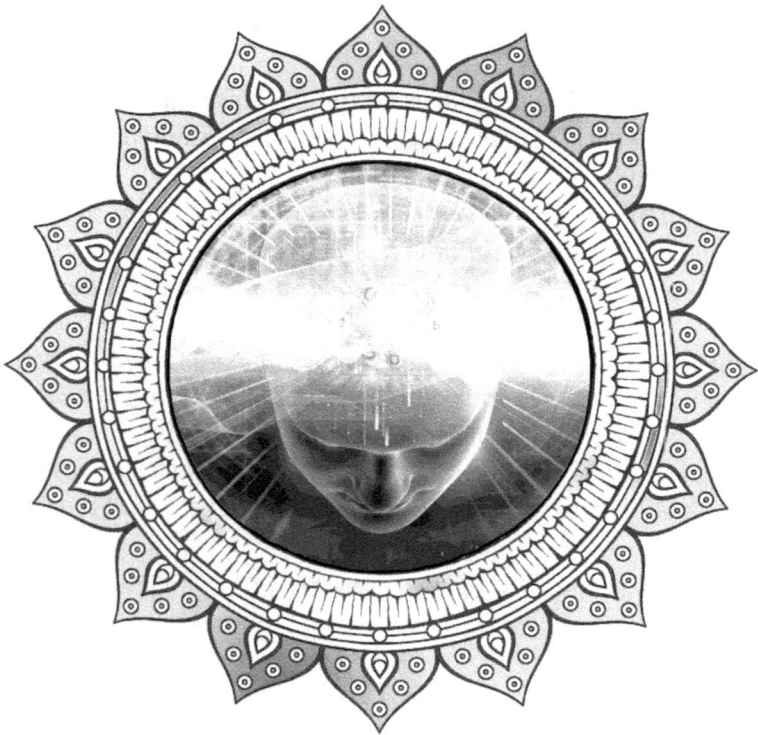

Runs My Body

End Pain

&

Feel Great Again!

Nineteen Proven Body, Mind, Spirit, and Fun Ways to Banish Pain Naturally

DUNCAN TOOLEY, CHI
Mind Trainer & Medical Hypnotherapist

Tooley Transformation Training Publications
2742 San Ramon Drive
Rancho Palos Verdes, CA 90275
310-832-0830   email: FeelGreat@duncantooley.com

FAIR USE NOTICE

DISCLOSURE

This book is for educational purposes and does not pretend to constitute the practice of medicine in any way. The techniques presented here are stand-alone and legal adjunct health-care, help-care wellness approaches and not the exclusive domain of any licensed healing arts profession. Many of the techniques presented are extremely popular because of their profound positive results. The author and publisher expressly disclaim responsibility for any adverse effects arising from the use, misuse, non-use, or application of the information contained in this book. You are a unique individual in your expression of mind-body-spirit. Use what is appropriate for you.

ACKNOWLEDGEMENTS

Thanks to Dr. Richard Steiner, Dr. Marita Pall, Dr. Leyla Ali, Janet Stanakis, Eva Margueriette, my family, and numerous friends for encouragement and editorial assistance. Special thanks to Dr. Shelley Stockwell-Nicholas, my teacher, mentor, coach, and friend in hypnosis and publishing. Acupressure diagram based on www.thetappingsolution.com. Artwork by the author with mandala images provided by Shelley Stockwell and students in my creative mandala classes.

ISBN: 0692691871
ISBN-13: 978-0692691878
Tooley Transformation Training Publications

DEDICATION

This book is dedicated to YOU, dear reader.
I wrote this for you and those you love.

As a Mind Trainer and
Medical Hypnosis Instructor,
I know that these tools,
plus your inherent powers
of body, mind, and spirit,
and your desire for fun
will transform your life so you feel great.

May the information and energy of this book
assist you to experience
your power
to heal yourself in every way.

Duncan

The circular image of a mandala
represents your wholeness
and your innate ability
to renew, restore, and regenerate.

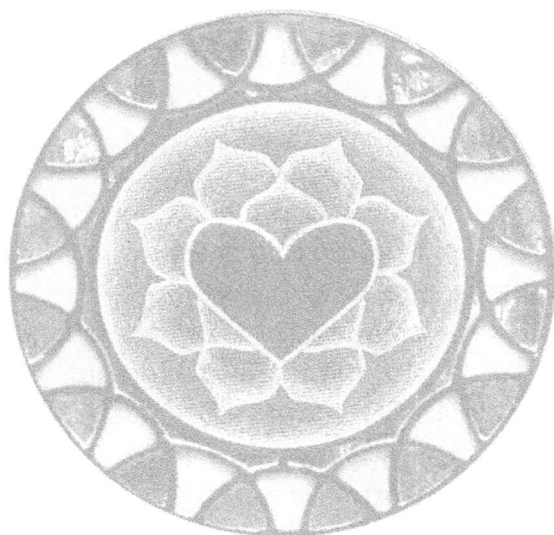

Let the energy of the mandalas in this book
remind you of your own power,
soak into your body,
heal any discomfort,
drain away any stress,
and bring you peace and joy!

Contents

x

Preface

Got pain? Would you rather feel great again? This book will show you how to turn that pain off! It is your easy step-by-step guide to rediscovery of your own power, and to relieve any discomfort you may experience, naturally without drugs. The methods are based on my own discovery experiences, those of my clients, and validation through medical studies. The following story illustrates the power available for you to access to feel great again.

My Miracle Story Begins

I had been working on software and computers (Information Technology) for 34 years when I started falling. I would just be walking along and suddenly I would fall. It started out slowly, maybe once every couple of weeks. Gradually it progressed to several times per week. Occasionally my hands would go totally numb while I was keyboarding. I went to see my normal doctor who immediately sent me to a neurologist. The neurologist stuck pins in different spots in my legs and feet and then ordered some nerve conduction tests. The tests were a series of electric shocks on various parts of my upper leg to simulate a nerve signal. Probes positioned on my foot measured the current. The attached computer calculated the speed and intensity of my nerve signal's movement from shock injection point to my foot. The same tests were conducted on my arms and hands.

The conclusion was clear: my nervous system was not functioning properly. My nerve signal propagation was weak and slow. The signal from my feet when I stepped on any unevenness in the ground surface was not getting to my brain fast enough. As a result, my brain's signal to muscles for a balance correction was not getting down to my legs in time. Down I went without any warning. Splat!

Neuropathy

The neurologist said I had *bilateral idiopathic peripheral neuropathy*. Neuropathy is loss of nerve function. Peripheral means that it was in my limbs and not in the brain or spinal column. Bilateral meant that I had it in both my right and left arms and legs. Idiopathic means *"we don't know the cause."* Diabetes or trauma is often the cause of neuropathy, but I had neither. I did have some burning sensation in my feet and they got numb and woke me from sleep. The solution offered was to begin taking Neurontin, live with it, and come back in a month for retesting (via sticking me with pins) to see if it was getting better or worse.

My colleagues at Computer Science Corporation were embarrassed by my random falls and concerned about the impression on clients. CSC put me on medical disability leave.

Every month I went back for the retest. The doctor said my condition was slowly getting worse. Specifically he said: "The good news is it won't kill you; the bad news is it may put you in a wheelchair." I researched neuropathy on my own and found that there are hundreds of variants, mostly of unknown origin, and some caused by a DNA mutation and limited to a family with that mutated gene. The probability was for a hereditary connection since I have an uncle with nondiabetic neuropathy.

Nerve Biopsy Is Like a Lightning Hit!

Finally I agreed to my doctor's suggestion that I had been resisting, a nerve biopsy in the Tulane University medical research hospital in New Orleans. The nerve doctor there made an incision in my left ankle, found the nerve to the top of my foot and cut it to get a sample for slides. DO NOT EVER AGREE TO A NERVE BIOPSY! It is like getting hit with a lightning bolt! I have been shocked by a car ignition system, (unplug a spark plug wire with the engine running) and the biopsy was about a hundred times worse!

I don't remember all the medical mumbo-jumbo of the report, but the microscope slide of the cross-section of the nerve bundle showed only a few nerves when it should have looked like the cross-section of a big underground telephone cable system with many, many conductors. This was not a hopeful report!

My neurologist kept up his monthly pin sticking and increase in my Neurontin until I finally agreed to go for the most advanced neurological diagnosis facility in the US, the Houston Methodist Hospital next to the famous M D Anderson Cancer Hospital. The 3-day intensive nerve system exam had helped thousands, and I had hopes of some new and better news for me.

Optimism

After the initial battery of tests that ruled out diabetes and some other causes on the first day, a group of doctors came to my room early on the second day. They were smiling and said that they had good news. They said, "There are some things that can relieve your neuropathy, but we need to complete all the tests before we give you the full report."

On the third day when they came back, the doctors were not smiling. They said, "Nondiabetic neuropathy is usually the result of either nerve death or sheath damage by an autoimmune system attack. But you have both causes: scarcity of cells and sheath damage!" Previously, they had been optimistic because they had found the sheath damage from my immune system, and there are treatments for that. Then they reviewed the slides I had transferred from Tulane and they saw the massive nerve cell death that left only a few remaining nerves. Now they said, "There is nothing that can be done about the nerve loss."

CIDP + Hopelessness

The lead doctor said that he was going to call my problem Chronic Inflammatory Demyelinating Polyneuropathy (CIDP) because that is a treatable problem that medical insurance would cover. He felt that it would be worth trying to get some relief from the autoimmune sheath damage part of the problem. He said he would not mention the scarcity of nerve cells because that is not treatable and would prevent insurance coverage of any treatment.

When my neurologist got the report, he began my treatment with a week of daily infusions of gamma globulin to boost my immune system. Gamma globulin is a dried powder concentrate of the immune system proteins from the blood of at least a thousand donors. The infusion procedure is to check into the hospital and wait for the solution of the powder into an infusible liquid. This preparation process takes at least an hour because if done too rapidly the solution foams. Since air bubbles must not be injected, slow mixing is the rule. Slow infusion follows, taking 6-8 hours to infuse the solution.

I did feel somewhat better after the week of infusions, so I was put on a program of 2 days of infusion once per month. The gamma globulin must have been having some good effect because it felt like an energy boost with the infusions that would gradually decline throughout the month. One month there was insufficient hospital supply of gamma globulin to infuse for two days, so I got one infusion in the beginning of the month and the second one halfway through the month when the hospital supply was restored. That worked better by giving two smaller energy spikes and declines. Thereafter, I did one infusion day in the hospital every other week.

Gamma Globulin + Neurontin + Methadone

Meanwhile, my primary care physician put me on daily methadone to aid the neuropathy pain. My routine of daily methadone, three daily doses of Neurontin, and biweekly gamma globulin infusions went on for over a year. Simultaneously, I noticed my mind would wander off into weird daydreams that had never happened before. When I mentioned this strange phenomenon to another neurologist at a health fair, he said: "Of course! Neurontin affects your nervous system. Where is the biggest concentration of your nervous system? In your brain." I went home and read all of the side effects of Neurontin. That's when I decided that the negatives outweighed the benefits and stopped taking it. I also stopped the methadone because the weekly hassle involved with getting it seemed to outweigh the benefits. Since methadone it is a controlled substance, I could only get a week's supply and had to go personally collect a new prescription from the physician each week. I continued the hospital infusions.

Go West

To understand what happened next, a little background is needed. Two factors converged:

1) I am a stained glass artist as a secondary career. I had a small business with a couple of employees fabricating the glass that I designed while I was off on my IT consulting assignments.

2) My wife, Dona, met a high school friend who had become a hypnotherapist. She helped Dona with a life-long problem so profoundly that Dona decided to become a hypnotherapist herself. Dona got certified and attended a conference for hypnotists in Detroit. At the conference, she met an instructor whose energy she liked and decided to take one of her classes in California.

Dona accepted my offer to accompany her to San Pedro, CA, from Baton Rouge, Louisiana, where we were living at that time. I called architects from our hotel room and promoted my stained glass business while she attended class each day.

Craziest Idea Ever!

One evening, Dona invited her instructor, Shelley Stockwell Nicholas, up to our room to meet me. Within minutes, she invited me to take her hypnosis class. My reaction was instantaneous: "That's the craziest idea I ever heard of! Why in the world would I ever want to take your class?" Without hesitation, Shelley fired back: "It will make you a better stained glass artist!" That overcame my resistance and got me thinking, "Well, maybe it could help and it probably can't hurt to find out." By the end of that week I had decided to return with Dona for the next hypnosis class in three months.

In my first hypnosis class I learned much that I had never heard before, but the most impressive fact was that *my mind was running my body.* As someone with a history of three disc ruptures, two back surgeries, an unknown strain of hepatitis, and now neuropathy, this was intriguing news! I had never heard any of this in my family or during my years of education. I also learned basic self-hypnosis. Dona and I decided that we should return to learn more in the next level hypnosis class.

My Pink Dilemma

Three months later, we are making our last-minute preparations to travel on the weekend to California for the Monday through Friday class when I discover my urine is the color of pink grapefruit juice! My doctor confirmed the presence of blood and gave me an order for a series of tests to determine the cause from a list of 25 possibilities. My problem is there is no time for these tests without canceling our trip until the next class, another three months in the future.

I have a real dilemma! I don't want to cancel the trip, and I don't want whatever is the cause to get worse, and I don't want to worry about it for the next 10 days until I can get back to take the tests! What to do? Then I remembered the important lesson from the first class, "Your subconscious mind is running your body." I realized what I had to do.

I used the self-hypnosis that I had learned to put myself into a relaxed state where my subconscious was more receptive. I gave myself this instruction: "Subconscious, because you run my body, I know that you know what is going on with this blood in my urine. I also know that you know how to fix it because the body is made to heal itself. I not only give you permission, but I COMMAND you to fix it NOW!"

My Miracle Story #1: I Learn To Cure Myself!

The next morning my urine was normal color. We went on our trip as planned. My urine continued to be normal in the following weeks. I never had the tests performed and I never went back to the doctor. Case closed! That is my first miracle story! I commented to Dona how powerful the whole experience was. Her response was, "Why don't you use that process on your neuropathy?" My reaction was, "Duh! I should have thought of that, but I didn't!"

Self-Hypnosis for Neuropathy

I made myself a CD of instructions to my nerve cells and immune system that I played as I fell asleep each night and first awoke in the morning. (These are the two most powerful times for infusing subconscious instructions because the conscious, resistant, critical mind is not fully present at those times.) The summary of the instructions was "Nerve cells, grow back. Don't worry that the doctors say you cannot! Just do it! Immune system, leave the nerve cells alone!"

My Miracle Story #2: I Cure Myself Again!

After doing this daily for about five weeks, I noticed that I was feeling better. I stopped the hospital infusions and still felt good. When my symptoms disappeared, I knew that again I had worked my own miracle of curing myself!

I have a scientist mentality, math and physics minors on my degree in secondary education, plus seven years teaching chemistry, math, and physics. My science mind wanted to understand what had happened. I found my answer in the many medical studies about the medical benefits of hypnosis. These studies document the ability of hypnosis to switch off pain and accelerate many types of healings. (See a partial list in *Appendix A6*).

The Moment of Decision

A deep emotional sense of loss swept over me. At 65 years, I had never heard about this power of the mind to transform the body. I suffered several back surgeries and the pain resulting from refusing the third surgery when I could have turned this pain off if I had known about this power. When I thought about the millions of people who suffer from back pain needlessly, I felt an urgency to help them discover, as I had, their power to heal themselves.

I decided to leave behind what I knew best, engineering computer systems. My future would be helping people use the power of their mind to get themselves well and happy. That day my career as a mind trainer and medical hypnotist began. With Dona, I registered for the next hypnosis class that would move me from master hypnotist to hypnotherapist. It was three months later during that class that the next miracle began.

What Is Deep Inside?

During the first day of class the instructor, Shelley, asked me while I was in trance, "If you could be doing anything in the world right now, what would you most like to be doing?" I answered, "Watching the sunset on the Pacific Ocean." The rest of the class turned and looked at Dona, who was utterly startled by my answer. I too was dumbfounded! I had never thought or expressed such a desire before.

I thought about that response over the next days. As I did, I detected some subconscious connections that had been below my awareness level. I associated love with the sun because the big orange sun was low on the horizon that moment when I really understood how much God loved me. It was the deep unconditional love of a woman that moved me. It was my very first love, not Dona, who expressed a depth of love that I had not experienced from my parents. It burned deep in my soul. For the first time I really knew that I was lovable and really, really loved! That orange sun got deeply imprinted along with that feeling of love.

And then there was my art. I had been painting sunsets and creating them in mosaics and stained glass. I did them just because I liked them, without realizing my spiritual connection deep inside. As Dona and I talked about the idea of moving to California to pursue our new hypnotherapy careers, that possibility seemed to grow. But what would it be like to move from our Louisiana roots to California? Where to live? What are the housing costs? Where do we start?

Shelly wanted to help us settle this issue since it was her question that stirred all this up. She was friends with a couple, Dr. Lilia and her husband, who were undecided about either selling or remodeling their house with a westerly ocean view. "Did we want to take a look to begin to get an idea about California housing?" We agreed, and so did the owners. The house was 50 years old and desperately in need of a remodel. There were big wrinkles in the aged carpet, black around the air ducts, and a tiny kitchen with ancient appliances, but the vast unobstructed ocean view was spectacular. The opportunity looked really interesting. We needed some references to gauge its value.

California Leaning

When the class was over on Friday, we contacted a real estate agent to show us some houses that overlooked the ocean. We didn't really like any of them, but we did get a good feel for the pricing of houses in the area. For homes in Louisiana, the land was usually about 1/5th of the total value of a home and the building 4/5ths. I learned that along the California coast, 4/5ths is the value of the land and 1/5th is the value of the house. By the end of the day I felt I had gathered sufficient reference points to make an offer on the spectacular-view home that needed the remodel.

Sunday morning Jon, Shelley's husband and former contractor, accompanied me to make our offer. Dona stayed with Shelley and was feeling very queasy about this plan. She said to Shelley, "I am 65. I think I'm getting too old for all this moving." To which Shelley responded, "You better make up your mind because Duncan is up there making an offer!"

When I made the offer to purchase the house, Dr. Lilia immediately said, "No!" It was not "let's talk," or a counter offer. In that instant my offer tipped the balance of indecision to remodel instead of sell. She realized that she would never find another house with such a spectacular view, and she was not ready to give it up.

Ready!

When I told Dona about the rejection of our offer, an involuntary tear began to roll down her cheek. Then she knew that she was ready to move to California! We left for the airport and the flight back to Louisiana thinking that we would be back in three months for the next class and more house-hunting. Meanwhile, we could do some Internet house-hunting before we returned.

It was Sunday, August 10, 2006, the day the airports began enforcing tighter security about liquids and other objects carried aboard airlines. We got to Los Angeles International airport hours early to allow for the expected delays. Everything went smoothly. I called my daughter to pick us up in New Orleans at midnight, as expected. Eventually our flight arrived. The incoming passengers were getting off the plane, and our bags were sitting on the tarmac waiting to be loaded for our flight home.

Don't Get On The Plane!

I got a cell phone call from Shelley who said, "Don't get on the plane! We found your house!" I began scratching my head and trying to figure out what to do next. I told Dona Shelley's message. Dona said, "Tell her you will call back.

Then, go tell the gate attendant that you have an emergency and can't get on the flight."

I did that and described the bags to the attendant who immediately radioed the baggage handlers, notated the change in the computer, and sent us down to baggage claim to retrieve our bags. She never asked what the emergency was, and the notation meant that we did not have a fee for changing our departure date. I called my daughter and left a message for her not to come to New Orleans to pick us up because our flight was canceled.

As we grabbed our two lonely bags off the conveyor belt, my daughter called back and asked, "Was it just your flight that was canceled, or were other flights also canceled?" She is concerned because of the new security issues. I admitted to her, "Actually we canceled our flight because we are going to stay a few more days." As I hung up, Dona said, "She is going to figure out that we are moving to Los Angeles!"

My Miracle Story #3:
The Universe Delivers Our Perfect House

While we had been waiting in the airport, Jon and Shelley had looked at an open house for sale to see if it met our specifications. Because it had no ocean view, it did not. They asked the real estate agent if he knew of a house for sale with an ocean view. He did, and directed them to a house a few blocks away. The house was unoccupied and not open, but it had an ocean view and an obvious remodel could be seen through the windows. This house met every one of the criteria we had developed, including Dona's wish that not a single remodel or update be required. Besides calling us, Shelley also called the real estate agent to meet us at the house.

We all met and inspected the house and property. The back yard contained a magnificent tree that formed a canopy over most of the yard. The elevation was 900+ feet and fell off steeply with unobstructed view to the ocean about 3 miles away. The property behind the house was owned by the city and unsuitable for development.

My Miracle Story #4: All Proceeds like Magic

Trusting the Universe that had led us this far, we signed an offer on the house the next day without even figuring out how we would finance it. From that moment, everything continued to proceed as if by magic. The owner, a woman in her 80's who had been the only occupant since the house was built in 1950, accepted our offer and had the contractor complete the few picky details that we insisted upon. The financing worked out better than expected with deposit refunds at closing. We stayed an additional week to get the house inspected and to initiate all the necessary paperwork for the purchase.

When we returned to Louisiana, our grown children found it difficult to believe that we had suddenly decided to move. Some suspected that we had been captured and brainwashed by a crazy California cult!

We asked them to expedite removal of their stored possessions from our attic because we were moving and planning to sell our Baton Rouge home. Some of the antique bedroom furniture what we had bought in Europe for each of our children was still in the attic. When several children said they were not ready to take their share, Dona's response was, "Pretend we have died and gone to California. We are selling the house empty. If you want your stuff, you have to take it now!"

We moved into our California dream house by mid-October, barely 70 days after the first hint of change. What followed was the normal getting settled and starting my business officially in February 2007. I continued my hypnosis studies. As I was completing my course in Hypnosis for Anesthesia, I discovered that I had an umbilical (belly button) hernia that needed surgical repair.

Walk Your Talk

I had always heard that you should *walk your talk.* I was becoming a hypnotist to assist people to use hypnosis for pain, even in place of anesthesia. I felt I needed to use hypnosis for my surgery so that I would personally have that experience. I planned on asking Shelley, my teacher, to hypnotize me in the operating room. When the surgeon nixed that plan because of hospital regulations about personnel in the operating room, I decided to do it myself with self-hypnosis.

My Miracle Story #5:
The Surgeon Can't Tell the Difference

The doctor agreed to permit me to use self-hypnosis for my anesthesia. To prepare for surgery, I wrote myself a script of walking across the sand at the beach into the ocean up to my chest. I imagined that the water was so cold that it numbed my body up beyond the surgery area, thereby keeping me totally comfortable during the surgery. After several practices with my miniature tape recorder to get the script right, I was ready!

In the hospital surgery prep area, the anesthesiologist asked me to sign a pink consent form that stated my acknowledgement that anything can go wrong, including death. I refused to sign it! I told her that I was not going to have general anesthesia; instead, I was going to use self-hypnosis. She flew into a screaming rage and stormed out.

A few minutes later she returned and said, "I have only one question. Do you want me in the operating room or not?" I answered: "Not." I think that was a question about pay.

Delay in the OR

In the operating room, the nurses asked me to delay starting my recorder with headphones until they had attached all their monitors to me. They forgot to tell me when they were finished and I could start! When I heard the surgeon scrubbing, I started my self-hypnosis script. It was too late! I was just walking across the sand in my imagination when I felt the pressure of the scalpel, but it didn't matter! My conviction that I would feel no pain made me totally comfortable, even though only lightly hypnotized.

The only part that was slightly uncomfortable was when the surgeon pulled the stitches tight. I then deliberately laughed to send some extra endorphins flooding into my brain.

When the surgeon and his assistant did the inventory of instruments, the assistant surgeon said to my surgeon, "I wasn't so sure that this guy was going to be able to put himself out like this." I was, of course, awake and aware, as you always are when hypnotized, so I thought this was a very funny statement. I spoke up and said, "You know guys, I am not really OUT. I'm just listening to everything you are saying." They didn't say much after that!

No Recovery. Go Home!

Because surgery recovery is about getting the anesthesia out of your body, there was no need for me to go to recovery. I was taken back to the surgery prep area. When the surgeon came to see me a few minutes later, I asked if I go, and was discharged within 30 minutes.

Because I used hypnosis, my wound healed rapidly with very little discomfort. I later shared an office with that surgeon until he retired. His testimonial that he could not tell the difference between me and a patient under the usual gas anesthesia is still available on my website: *www.DuncanTooleyHypnosis.com/hypnosis-effectiveness-reviews.* Why he risked his reputation, letting a relative stranger to do his own anesthesia, is another part of this miracle.

More Miracles

During the next eight years, I witnessed many more miracles. They were the miracles that my clients created in themselves by using their power of mind. I witnessed clients shrink their stomach as if they had a surgical gastric band by using a "Mental Gastric Band®" with the power of their imagination. I heard heavy drinkers and smokers say "It was like magic!" when they kicked their addiction through visualization and positive self-talk.

I shared the joy of those who got their life back through use of techniques in this book after unsuccessfully trying many other remedies for chronic pain. I witnessed the birth of two grandchildren without drugs, pain, or strain when my daughter used self-hypnosis. I have come to believe that what others might call "miracles" are what we are naturally meant to accomplish through the power of our mind with its deep connection to the SuperMind, the Infinite, the Divine.

My Miracle Story #6: I Repair My Heart Valve

In 2010 I had a few moments where my speech did not match the words I was trying to say. The doctors called it a possible TIA (Transient Ischemic Attack, or mini-stroke), which left no evidence. A small amount of turbulence was detected in my heart that was not considered related. I simply told my body to keep on working perfectly.

After Dona died in 2015, I got my heart checked as part of getting myself in top shape for my next segment of life. An echocardiogram showed a malformed mitral valve that the cardiologist rated *moderate leaning toward severe* and immediately wanted to replace the valve. Instead, I told him that I choose to care for it through hypnosis, my body's natural healing forces powered by a positive, believing mind. He agreed to a recheck in nine months. I told him that the results were going to show an improved heart valve. He replied, "That's not possible!"

In April 2016, I had been talking to the cells in my body for nine months, encouraging them to be happy and well and perfect. I was so certain of valve improvement that I informed my family about the forthcoming echocardiogram miracle evidence a week before the test was to be done.

Sure enough, the new echocardiogram showed that the valve was only moderately malformed with no action needed. My cardiologist confirmed the improvement by comparing the old and new images side-by-side. I continue to talk to my cells every morning and evening and feel younger and younger with each new day.

Why the Miracle Stories?

Here is what I learned though the events recounted in these stories:

- We all have a very powerful mind that controls every aspect of our body, and it seems somehow able to draw upon awesome, even infinite, power.
- Our thoughts and intentions have a powerful effect on ourselves, on people and circumstances so that magic and miracles seem to happen automatically.

The important message for YOU from these miracle stories:

- *You have the identical same power.*
- *You can work your own miracles with the same tools!*

Book Organization

We are on this earth-walk to have fun as a body-mind-spirt life-form. (Cf. *Appendix A2. Mind-Body-Spirit Model*).

Hence, the book organizes the relief and feel great again methods into the categories of ***body, mind, spirt,*** and ***fun***.

Each method begins with an ***About*** explanatory introduction and is then detailed in easy-to-follow ***Steps*** (or options). An occasional ***Story*** or ***Study*** illustrates or reinforces the content of a technique. Some stories have the client's name included with permission; others have the names changed or omitted. ***Pro-Tips*** are included on some techniques as suggestions for a deeper mastery. ***Extras*** are references to useful auxiliary material on the book website *www.feelgreat.duncantooley.com*.

The APPENDICES section contains related information for the curious, including some answers to *why* and *how* these 19 pain-relieving methods work. The REFERENCES section contains the list of books I consulted in assembling those few parts of the content that were not from my direct experience, as well as the sources for referenced studies.

If you are using this material as a caregiver, or to assist another, the techniques that best serve another's needs may differ from those you would select for yourself.

You can help others by permitting me to tell your success story with these methods in future editions. Please email me your success story from using these methods; email to *feelgreat@duncantooley.com*. I also welcome your feedback and comments on social media.

Thank you for sharing your invaluable experiences and inspiration to help others!

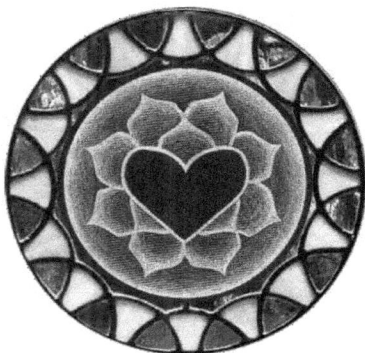

Introduction . . . About Pain

The REIGN of PAIN is mainly in the BRAIN!

Fundamental Truth

Your brain cannot tell the difference between your perception of an experience and the actual physical experience. What you tell your mind, your mind believes.

Your mind gets input from three sources:
- Your senses
- Your memory
- Your imagination

Your mind treats the information from all three inputs equally. Your mind cannot tell the difference between senses, memory, and imagination.

19

You have the power to direct your imagination any way you choose. As a result, you are able to take control of the effects of your memory and your senses with your imagination and turn off pain. It is this power of your imagination, working with the physiology of your body, that is the basis for the techniques in this book.

This book is for you if you experience any kind of pain. You don't have to own the pain, so I avoid calling any discomfort "your" pain.

Physiology of Your Nervous System

The nervous system of your body is composed of the central nervous system (the brain and spinal cord), the peripheral nervous system (the sensory and motor neurons), and the autonomic nervous system (which regulates body processes such as digestion and heart rate). The processes in this book will assist you to train your brain to interpret information from your nervous system in the way that makes you feel great!

Brain and Pain

Your brain is the endpoint of the relay system that is the pain network. When a peripheral nerve fires, the signal is passed to the nerves in the spinal cord. The information is processed there and passed to the brain stem. Part of the spinal cord processing may involve firing a motor nerve cell to stimulate a muscle contraction to move the affected area away from the pain source.

The information passed to the brain stem goes to the mid-brain region. From there it is analyzed and may be sent to the cortical brain region, specifically that area that has come to be known as the brain's *pain center*. It is at that point that you *feel* the pain.

Pain As Interpretation

Something is happening in the body, and your brain applies meaning and triggers emotion to interpret what is going on. This means that if your brain did not interpret, then there would be no pain! The pain occurs only after the circuit is completed by the brain's interpretation of the signal.

Consider how many times you may have cut yourself without realizing it. Perhaps it was a paper edge or a sharp blade you were using. Most likely it did not hurt until you *saw* the blood, possibly minutes or more after the cut actually happened! This shows your brain's role in interpreting what it believes *should be* pain.

How to Stop Pain?

The three methods for stopping the sensation of pain all focus around preventing the nerve stimulation signal from reaching that bundle of brain neurons that is identified as the pain center:

1. **Stop the nerve stimulation at its source**. This stops the peripheral nerve cells from firing. In its simplest form this is something like: "Take your hand out of the fire!"

   Local anesthetics are also in this category. They chemically bind to nerve cells and prevent them from producing nerve signals.

2. **Block the signal from reaching the brain.** Neurons sensitive to vibration, temperature, and pressure transmit at a faster rate than pain neurons. Therefore, it is possible to flood the neural pathway with other nerve sensations so that the pain signal gets blocked or overpowered.

21

When you instinctively rub a painful area or apply heat or cold to "relieve" the pain, what you are doing is blocking the pain signal from reaching your brain by flooding the neural relay system with other information. (Epidural injections and nerve blocks also operate by this method of blocking the pain signal from reaching your brain. They are listed here for information and not as a recommendation).

3. **Prevent the signal from reaching the pain center.** Even though the nerve signal has arrived in your brain, you do not feel the sensation of discomfort until your brain processes it and sends it to the *pain center.* This method prevents the signal from being *interpreted* as pain by stimulating other parts of your brain instead of the pain center. Most of the techniques in this book work like this. (See my initiation to awareness of this interpretation effect in Appendix *A5. Interpretation Revelation*).

Call Pain by Its Proper Name!

There is nothing either good or bad, but thinking makes it so. - Hamlet 2, 2

Pain is mostly named from a time perspective: *acute,* short term, and *chronic*, long term. Sometimes we call pain *good pain* or *bad pain.* However, from your brain's perspective, what counts is the purpose and intelligence conveyed by the discomfort. From your brain's point of view, pain is either *informational* or *nuisance.*

Informational pain signals that something is not as it should be and needs attention. Informational pain is giving your mind, INFORMATION. Listening to your body provides information about the cause of discomfort, so that you can choose an appropriate response.

Nuisance pain is just that, a useless nuisance. Nuisance pain adds no value by its continuation after you have taken whatever measures you can to remedy what the informational pain was reporting. Not only does this pain have no value, it often adds debilitating stress.

Use the techniques in this book to relieve *nuisance* pain. If discomfort continues to get your attention, the discomfort you experience may still be *informational*, calling you to learn more from your body. Begin now to learn to discern from the techniques in this book what is *informational pain* and what is *nuisance pain* for you.

Story: My client, Glen, suffered a ruptured vertebra disc while alone at work. He couldn't get off the floor until he used my *60-Second Turn Down* method (Chapter 2). Later he told me it would have been impossible to drive to the hospital had he not used that method to lower his experience of pain.

Analysis: Since Glen had accepted the informational value of the pain, ("Something in my back needs attention!"), and had decided upon a remedial action ("Get to the hospital!"), it was appropriate to convert his *informational* pain experience into a *nuisance* pain that he could turn off. Even though nothing about the firing of his neurons had changed, he transformed his discomfort into a *nuisance* by his remedial action and his decision to ignore the pain. Notice that the difference between *informational* and *nuisance* pain is in your brain, not in the pain source.

My Story: My right knee was screaming when I walked, so I went to my physician to have it checked. I used that *informational* pain to seek the appropriate remedial action, if any. An MRI revealed the jagged edge of a torn meniscus. The doctor recommended surgery to trim off the jagged edge.

When I decided not to do the surgery, that decision effectively converted my *informational* pain to *nuisance* discomfort. The original pain had done its job and now it was just a nuisance that I could ignore. I used the *Affirmations* method (Chapter 11) on my knee. Since then it has been very comfortable, only reminding me of its presence after *extreme* activity.

Caution!

Just because you learn the methods to interpret a discomfort as a nuisance and remove it from your perception doesn't mean that this is the best thing for you to do. You must make the personal decision about what is in your best interest in each case. Only you know what is normal and OK for your body to endure. Be careful; be safe; listen to your body's information. Decide wisely when to consider discomfort a nuisance and turn it off via the methods in this book, and when to consider it information that you must continue to investigate.

Many athletes turn off or ignore informational pain. Often they suffer permanent injuries as a result.

> ***Story:*** Famous baseball player Lou Gehrig played 2,130 consecutive baseball games despite broken fingers. When Gehrig's hands were X-rayed late in his career, doctors spotted 17 different fractures that had *healed* while Gehrig continued to play. Gehrig had decided to ignore, 17 times, the informational pain from his broken fingers. He decided to consider the pain as nuisance pain and used his mind to ignore it.

Your Mantra

*"I discern whether my discomfort is **Informational** or **Nuisance**.*
*If **Informational**, I listen and take appropriate action.*
*If **Nuisance**, I turn it off."*

Extra: Print six reminder cards with your mantra from the book extras website: *www.feelgreat.duncantooley.com*

Practical & Easy Techniques

This book contains 19 step-by-step techniques that utilize some aspect of your nervous system, brain, and mind to conquer pain and provide easy pain relief. Each technique will assist you to feel comfortable and pain-free quickly, and perhaps permanently, so you feel great again. The techniques can be used individually or in combination for even greater and longer-lasting relief. Your mind-body-spirit combination is unique to you and like no other.

Enjoy letting the 19 techniques work their marvelous effect as you determine YOUR best relief process and discover YOUR favorites among the methods presented.

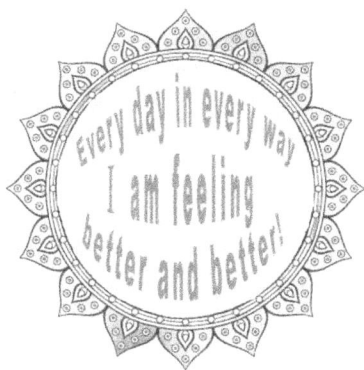

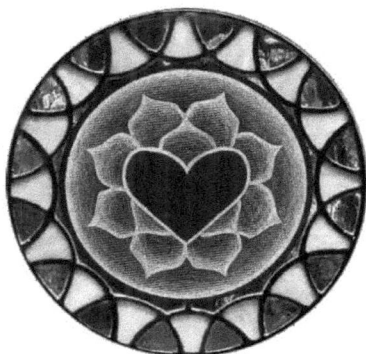

BODY-BASED METHODS TO FEEL GREAT AGAIN

▶ *1. Talk to Your Cells*

▶ *2. Tooley 60-Second Turn Down*

▶ *3. Temperature-Pressure-Vibration*

▶ *4. Relaxation Response*

▶ *5. Acupressure*

▶ *6. TENS*

▶ *7. Physical Exercise*

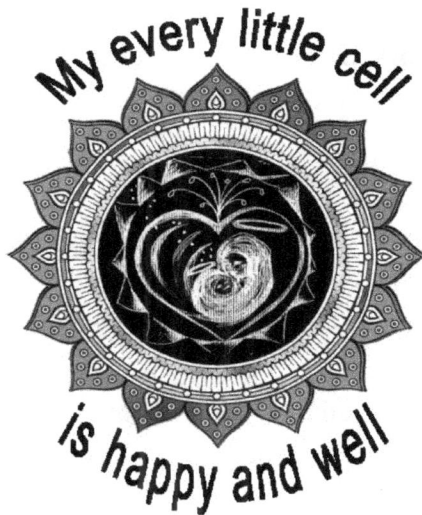

Chapter 1

My every little cell is happy and well

Talk To Your Cells

"Talk to the pain. Tell the subconscious: 'Give it up! Reveal the emotions so I can deal with and dissipate them'." – Dr. Scott Brady

About Talk to Your Cells

The cells in your body have intelligence and know what they are supposed to do. Each one carries the blueprint for your whole being. However, external environmental factors, your internal beliefs, and your emotions modify the expression of the genetic instructions through the epigenetic switches in your DNA. This technique is based upon interacting consciously with the intelligence of your cells by both questioning and instructing.

Steps to Use Talk to Your Cells

Step 1. Ask Your Cells What Is Going On in Your Body.

Your cells know what is happening in your body. They are the causes and participants in your sensations. They know your physical situation far better than anyone else can diagnose. Use your *Relaxation Response* (Chapter 4) to get yourself into the relaxed state. Then ask your cells:

- "What is going on?"
- "What is the cause of this specific discomfort?"
- "Why are you getting my attention?"
- "Is this discomfort Informational or Nuisance?"
- "What action do you want me to take?"

After you ask each question, pay attention to the first thought that pops into your mind. That is the way the cells communicate their intelligence to you (besides triggering the nervous system). Pay attention to that first thought; don't reject, judge, censor, or ignore it. Take that first thought as your answer, even if you don't understand it. You can ask for clarification, if needed, after you have your answer.

Step 2. Follow the Advice/Instruction from Your Cells.

This information comes from your connection to the Super-Conscious, the timeless and divine wisdom of the ages. Heed it!

> *Story:* My client Lisa said, "I am going to the hospital emergency room when I finish lunch because my menstrual bleeding has been abnormal for more than 2 weeks." I suggested that we do a hypnosis session first. In trance, I had her ask her All-Wise, All-Knowing

aspect of herself (her Super-Conscious), "Is it in my best interest to check into the emergency room?"

The answer she got was, "No! Western doctors have no answers for you. You need to go to a good Chinese herbalist and follow her instructions."

When she came out of the trance, her question for me was, "What is an herbalist? Where did that come from? That's not a word in my vocabulary! I don't know what it means!"

She went to an herbalist, took the recommended herbs, and is now better!

Step 3. Tell Your Cells What You Desire.

Overcome any cellular confusion by talking to your cells. Give them clear instructions about your desires. Consider your instructions as altering your DNA, because in fact that is what you are doing. You are altering the expression of specific genes by flipping the epigenetic switches of your DNA through your belief-backed speech.

Tell your cells how much you appreciate the work they do for you. Talk to the cells in that area of your body that is uncomfortable and tell them: "Relax! Be comfortable! Be well!" Use whatever words you find most meaningful to speak to your cells.

> *My Story:* One morning I noticed that my urine was pink, resembling pink grapefruit juice. When my doctor confirmed that I had blood in my urine, and told me to schedule tests to determine the cause from among the 25 possibles, I didn't. Instead, I talked to my cells and cleared the problem, whatever it was. (See the story in the Preface under *My Pink Dilemma*).

> *Story:* Danielle, my adult daughter, had a pain in her hip that nagged her for almost a year, causing discomfort walking and difficulty sleeping. Several doctors unsuccessfully looked for an explanation and remedy.

Out of desperation, she began talking to her hip. She said:

> *"Nerve, if you are somehow pinched, move around and get yourself into a comfortable un-pinched position. Hip, figure out whatever is going on down there, and do whatever it takes to get yourself comfortable. I have work to do and I need for you to be comfortable, so get on with it."*

She repeated these same instructions, sometimes with slight variations, every day. A month later she noticed that she had no pain. She has not had a recurrence since.

Story: In the children's book *Good-Bye Bumps!*, Saje Dyer recounts the story from her childhood when her father, Wayne Dyer, suggested she talk to her long-standing face bumps (probably acne). The story recounts how she talked to her bumps and they went away.

Study: In a trial with 93 spinal surgery patients at the University of California (Davis) Medical Center, those who received specific instructions about blood flow lost about half as much blood compared to the controls and a third group taught another technique. The physician instructed preoperative patients: "Tell your blood to move away from the surgery site." (Cf. Study References, Study 1)

Notice the simplicity of the instructions given to the patients and the absence of procedures and detailed wording. The instruction was simple and brief: ask certain cells for a specific action. Implied in the simple command is belief that the cells have sufficient intelligence to know HOW they are to accomplish the action requested.

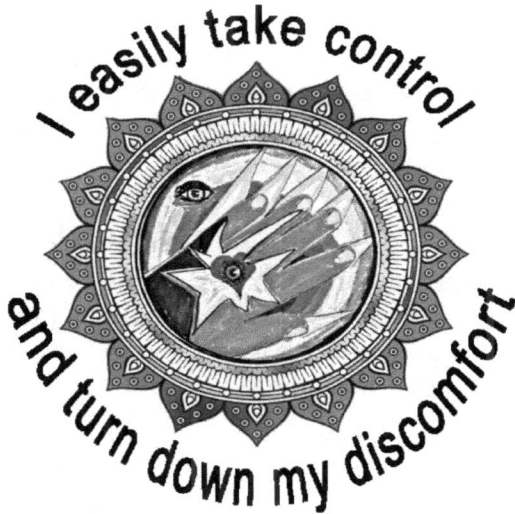

Chapter 2

Tooley 60-Second Turn Down

About Tooley 60-Second Turn Down

This technique uses the power of your imagination. It is quick, simple, easy to remember, and very effective. Your subconscious mind accepts imagination in the same way that your subconscious accepts the information coming in through your senses. Nearly everyone experiences significant relief with this turn-down process. Consider it your first line of offense for feeling better. At least 50%

pain reduction is usual, and many achieve 100% removal of discomfort.

If you have someone who can assist you for the first time, that's even better. Your assistant can lead you through the process so you can perform the simple steps with your eyes closed from the beginning. If you are doing the technique by yourself, memorize the steps first and then perform them with your eyes closed.

Steps to Use Tooley 60-Second Turn Down

1. Choose only one area of your body that is causing discomfort. Measure your discomfort intensity on a scale of 1-10, where 1 is very low and 10 is most intense. Remember the number.

2. Close your eyes, take a deep breath, and imagine the discomfort area as a shape, any shape. Give the shape a color (or a smell if you prefer).

3. Change the shape to some other shape then change the color (or smell) to another color (or smell). Change the shape and color slowly two more times.

4. Imagine a round volume control knob with the numbers 0 through 11 around the edge. Place the knob on top of your final shape, with the arrow pointing to the number of your discomfort level from the first step. Reach in and grab the knob and slowly turn it *UP* one number, making the pain intensity higher than your starting number, only for a moment.

5. When you feel your discomfort increase, turn the control back down to where you started. Slowly turn the knob down one number at a time, pausing on each number until the discomfort decreases on each step down. You can stop wherever you

choose, or you can continue to turn the knob and decrease the discomfort all the way down to zero.

Congratulations! That was great! Good job!

Notice how comfortable you feel! Amazing, isn't it! You have taken control and now you feel much better! You used your mind to control your body! You can always do this exercise to feel great!

Why this technique works

If pain happens to you, you can easily feel like a victim. In the *Tooley 60-Second Turn Down* process, you gradually take control back from pain and restore your power as you move from "victim" to "controller." First you take artistic control with the shape and color. Then you take intensity control with the "volume" knob adjustments.

PAIN, of itself, never really had any power. Whatever power pain seemed to have, you gave to it by surrendering *your* power over interpretation of what is happening in your body. With this turn-down process you affirm your power to interpret body sensations however you choose! You re-frame your experience from "victim" of discomfort to being a powerful "controller" of how you feel.

Story: When I was a presenter at a health fair, I used the 60-Second Turn Down technique with a man who said his pain level was a "10." At the end of the process his pain level was "0"! He called me a "Miracle Worker." I reminded him that HE is the miracle worker because he used the power of his mind to change his perception of pain. I assisted by supplying the technique that showed him how to do it.

Story: At a different wellness event, a woman came up to me on crutches. "I have a very painful heel spur," she said. When I asked her, "Would you like to reduce the pain level?" she answered "Yes, my pain level is 10." I instructed her to sit down and then used the *60-Second Turn Down* technique with her. After she opened her eyes and stood up, she exclaimed "The pain is gone! I can't believe it!" She went off carrying her crutches, looking for her husband to tell him.

Story: A client to whom I had taught the *60-Second Turn Down* technique had a dramatic back pain episode while alone at work. He later told me, "Using your technique allowed me to turn down my pain level enough so I could drive myself to the hospital. Before I used it, I was unable to get up off the floor."

Story: A participant in a cancer support services meeting told me she was suffering with pain. I used my *60-Second Turn Down* technique after the meeting with her. When I saw her a month later, she told me that she had successfully used the process many times for relief. She prevailed upon the administration of the cancer support center to add instruction about this technique to their curriculum of services.

Pro-Tip: If you are assisting someone in decreasing their discomfort by reading the instructions to them, be certain to include these important steps:

• Increase the pain level by turning the control knob *UP* one digit. This is the key empowering step because once a person experiences that the pain actually increases when they turn the knob up (and they will experience an increase!), they realize that they are able to control the discomfort sensation. The increase becomes the powerful convincer that they can decrease pain by turning the knob down!

• Offer to stop at intensity level 3, and level 2, and level 1. Initially the person you are assisting may not be able to believe that they can turn pain down lower than a level 3 or 2 or 1. The option of stopping at one of these levels permits the person to solidify the experience of lowering discomfort without violating their core beliefs. With subsequent uses they may be able to go lower.

Most who go for turning their discomfort down to level "0" (no discomfort) succeed in reaching it. They achieve level zero because, as they feel the discomfort decrease, they release any doubt of their ability to reach level zero. The power of their belief that they are in control makes complete relief a reality for them.

Extra: Get the Tooley *60-Second Turn Down* process written as a script to be used with another person. Get a friend to use it with you. Download and print from the book extras website: *www.feelgreat.duncantooley.com*

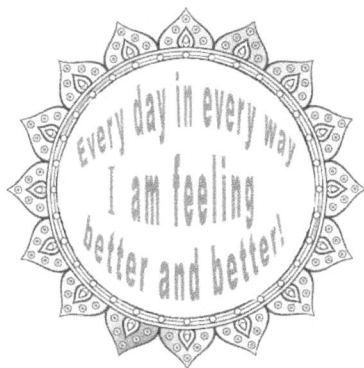

Chapter 3

Appropriate heat or cold makes me feel great

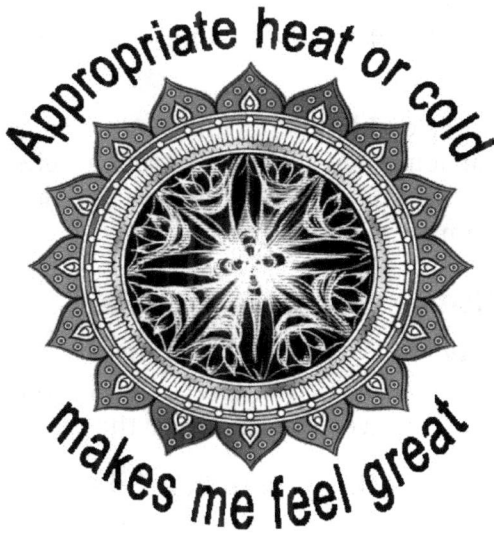

Temperature-Pressure-Vibration

About Temperature

Application of heat or cold relieves muscle discomfort. Signals from the temperature-sensitive neurons flood your nerve communication highway and block out signals from the pain-sensitive neurons.

Cold reduces swelling and inflammation, which helps prevent further discomfort from tissue damage. Ice packs are a standard pain-relieving tool present at all sporting events. Consumer freezer packs containing a gel that remains flexible below freezing temperatures are available in several shapes in cloth-wrapped bags with Velcro straps. The long narrow shape is suitable for use around the neck and around arms or legs. The large square shape is designed for the back, thighs, or other large areas.

Warmth speeds up blood flow and can promote healing by speeding nutrients and specialized repair cells to the site. Heating pads are inexpensive items to have ready in your arsenal to combat nuisance discomfort.

Steps to Use Temperature for Relief

Step 1. Apply Ice Pack to Painful Area.
Always protect the skin from direct contact with the ice by a layer of fabric between the skin and the ice.

Step 2. Apply Heating Pad to Painful Area.
Always protect the skin from direct contact with the heating pad by a layer of fabric between the skin and the pad.

Step 3. Combine with Pressure and/or Vibration
Temperature, pressure, and vibration applied to the painful areas utilize the same nervous system extensions of your brain as the neurons that transmit pain. These three techniques are simple and probably very familiar. They are included as reminders that they are part of our mind's available relief tools.

> *Pro-Tip:* My chiropractor says to apply cold first because cold will reduce the inflammation and stop the damage. Later, if the discomfort continues, apply the heat to accelerate the repair and to provide warming comfort.

Pro-Tip: Get a set of inexpensive freezer gel ice packs and keep them in your freezer to have them ready and available.

Pro-Tip: Get a heating pad to have ready and available.

~◻~◻~◻~

About Pressure

Overloading your nerve network with pressure can provide a big relief! Slower attention-getting discomfort signals get left behind and blocked.

A compression wrapping or elastic sleeve on the knees (knee wrap or brace) relieves or "prevents" knee discomfort because the signals from the pressure neurons continue to signal and arrive in the brain before any signals from the pain receptors. This is why squeezing or rubbing a stubbed toe is such a relief.

Tight bindings on wounds that prevent bleeding also reduce discomfort. Massage therapy applies pressure to loosen tight muscles and can be a source of relief.

Steps to Use Pressure for Relief

Step 1. Apply Continuous Pressure.

Apply a wrapping of gauze, Ace bandage, even duct tape! Take care that any wound dressing is sterile and the pressure still permits blood circulation.

Step 2. Remove the Need for Discomfort Relief.

Take necessary action to relieve the cause of the discomfort so that the pressure is no longer needed or useful.

Step 3. Get a Massage.

A massage with emphasis on the uncomfortable area can bring relief. Carefully explain to your masseuse what you desire, the pressure level, and what areas need attention. During the massage, let your masseuse know if any action is uncomfortable for you.

> ***My Story:*** The torn meniscus of my right knee sometimes causes discomfort. An elastic knee sleeve that applies pressure all around the knee increases comfort. I believe that the pressure closes the pain neuron gates as well as holds the meniscus in place.

~◻~◻~◻~

About Vibration

Vibration floods the sensory channels and overloads them so that the pain neuron signals don't reach the brain. Thus, vibration is similar in effect to temperature and pressure. Hand-held, battery-operated vibrator-massagers are convenient and inexpensive for relieving little annoyances all over the body. They are particularly useful for relieving neck tension from improper head position while sleeping or to relieve stress tension in the neck or shoulders.

Athletic whirlpools are portable tanks of water that spray high-powered jets of water, creating a vibratory massage effect in the entire tank in which the injured athlete sits. Whirlpools combine the effect of pressure and vibration. When hot water is used, the temperature effect is added, forming a near complete block of signals from the sensitive neurons. Jet sprays in Jacuzzis and bathtubs accomplish the same effect for non-athletes.

The Trans-cutaneous (across-the-skin) Electrical Nerve Stimulator (TENS) is a relief device based on electrical vibration to disrupt nerve signals. The *TENS* technique in Chapter 6 successfully relieved my substantial back strain. Be sure to read Chapter 6.

Steps to Use Vibration for Relief

Step 1. Use A Vibrator.

Get a hand-held, battery-operated vibrator-massager and use it.

Step 2. Use an Alternative Vibration Source.

If a vibrator is not available, create your own alternative vibration by rhythmically tapping or beating against that area of your body in discomfort.

Vibration speakers are small devices that vibrate a metal plunger that converts any object on which it is placed into a vibrating speaker. These are used as amplifiers for cell phone speakers and can be used as a source for relief vibration.

> *My Story:* The Tooley *Think Myself Slim* Mental Gastric Band Weight Loss program uses a vibration device (vibrator, speaker, or cell phone) as a sensory aid. The vibrator is placed over the area of the stomach where the weight loss client will squeeze their stomach wall muscles to create a simulated gastric band. The vibration assists the client in focusing their contraction energy on the specific muscles for the desired effect.
>
> A free introduction and sample of the program is available in my store: *store.duncantooley.com*

Chapter 4

Comfort flows over me as I relax more and more

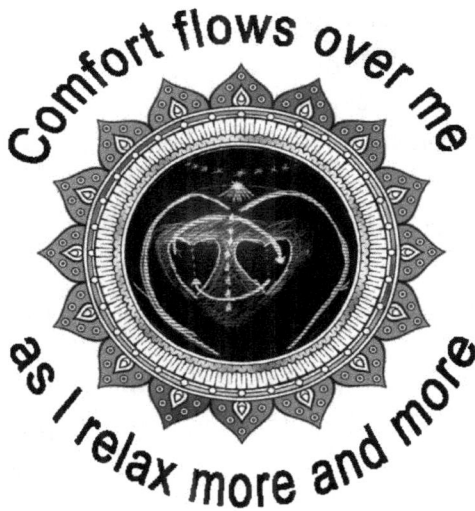

Relaxation Response

About the Relaxation Response

The Relaxation Response is your personal ability to cause your body to release chemicals and produce brain signals that make your muscles and organs slow down and increase blood flow to your brain. The Relaxation Response is a mentally active process that leaves your body relaxed. Like most techniques, it gets more effective with practice.

The National Institutes of Health (NIH) recognizes the Relaxation Response as having these broad health benefits:

- Reduction of pain
- Increased energy
- Decreased fatigue
- Improved sleep
- Lowered stress hormone levels
- Lowered blood pressure
- Increased motivation, productivity, and decision-making

The most popular methods for invoking the Relaxation Response are:

- Deep Breathing   (this chapter)
- Muscle Tensing/Relaxing (this chapter)
- Imagery   (this chapter)
- Hypnosis   (chapter 13)
- Meditation   (chapter 15)
- Yoga   (chapter 16)

All of these methods work. Which ones will you use? Sample each and decide for yourself the ones you like best. Below are detailed steps for the first three on the list. Separate technique chapters are devoted to several of the other methods.

~◻~◻~◻~

About Deep Breathing

Deep Breathing is the easiest element of relaxation and one of the most powerful. Because it is so powerful, it has become the first step in almost every healing modality. There are numerous breathing patterns; here are four:

Option A. Equal Breathing Pattern.

How it's done: Inhale to a count of four. Then exhale to a four count. Breathe all through the nose, which adds a natural resistance to the breath. After mastery, increase to 6 or 8.

Option B. Four-Square Breathing Pattern.

How it's done: The breath cycle has four equal parts (imagine going around a square track as you breathe). Inhale for a count of 4. Hold your breath for a count of 4. Exhale for a count of 4. Rest between breaths for a count of 4.

Option C. Abdominal Breathing Pattern.

How it's done: With one hand on the chest and the other on the belly, take a deep breath in through the nose, ensuring the diaphragm (not the chest) inflates with enough air that you feel your belly push your hand out. Fill your lungs at the end of the inhale. On the exhale, push your belly back toward your spine as far as you can, and then empty your lungs last. Take 6 to 10 deep, slow breaths per minute.

Option D. Alternate Nostril Breathing.

How it's done: With your right hand, extend your middle and index fingers and place them on your third eye (center forehead). Use your thumb and ring finger to alternately press lightly on the side of your nose and seal off one nostril and then the other. Follow this pattern:

1) *Seal left nostril with ring finger.*
2) *Inhale through right nostril.*
3) *Remove ring finger seal on left nostril.*
4) *Seal right nostril with thumb.*
5) *Exhale through left nostril.*
6) *Inhale through left nostril.*
7) *Remove thumb seal on right nostril.*
8) *Seal left nostril with ring finger.*
9) *Exhale through right nostril.*
10) *Repeat cycle, beginning with step 1.*

Balance your inhalations and exhalations so they are the same length through both nostrils. Repeat up to 10 full cycles, gradually increasing the number of repetitions as you gain experience. Always begin changes slowly, being sensitive to your body.

~◻~◻~◻~

About Muscle Tensing/Relaxing

Everyone has a resting level of muscle tension, some more than others. When you are under acute stress, your muscles have a higher level of resting tension that is fatiguing, and sometimes even painful. After you tense and relax muscles, the residual tension will drop below the original level.

Steps to Use Muscle Tensing/Relaxing for Relief

Step 1. Get Comfortable.

Sit, recline, or lie down. You can keep your eyes open or closed; most people prefer to close their eyes. If you are wearing glasses or contact lenses, you may be more comfortable by removing them before starting the exercise.

Step 2. Breathe Deeply and Slowly.

Begin to breathe deeply and slowly. Continue this deep breathing for at least one minute before moving to step 3.

Step 3. Progressive Tensing/Relaxing Muscle Groups.

Do a strong (but not painful) tensing for 2 or 3 seconds. Use your brain to focus on how the tension feels. Take a deep breath and on the exhale let all the tension go, saying "RELAX" as you feel the tension flow out of your body. Begin with your feet, while continuing to breathe deeply and regularly. Focus on the sensations of relaxation before moving to the next muscle group. Progress though these groups:

- Feet and toes
- Calves and thighs
- Hips and stomach
- Fingers and hands
- Lower and upper arms
- Back
- Shoulders and neck
- All the muscles in your face and jaw

Step 4. Finish the Exercise.

- Become aware of your surroundings (location, people, and noises).
- Move your feet, legs, hands, arms, and rotate your head.
- Open your eyes if they were closed.
- Notice the feeling of re-energized, refreshed, and relaxed.

Pro-Tip: Use parts of the tense-then-relax exercise in a shorter format when you need a quick relaxation break. For example, when sitting in traffic, you can get a burst of relaxation by tensing the muscles in your shoulders and upper back and then relaxing them.

~ロ~ロ~ロ~

About Imagery

In the Imagery technique you imagine experiences that are so captivating, so rich in detail, and so all-consuming, that you get lost in them and are distracted from everything else. This creates the Relaxation Response. This imagery is not only visual stimulation, but a complete sensory experience that involves sounds, aromas, tastes, tactile touch-sensations, and emotional feeling.

Steps to Use Imagery for Relief

Step 1. Relax.

Start the exercise by sitting or lying in a comfortable position. Relax and do a few minutes of deep breathing.

Step 2. Imagine Your Pleasant Place.

This time the focus is not on muscles but on a pleasant image in your mind. It's best to start with the image of a familiar favorite place, like your favorite place outdoors in nature, for example. Wherever you choose, make sure your choice is a peaceful and calming place. Use your full imagination with something for each of your senses.

For example, if imagining a place in the woods, in your mind:

- *See* the moss, the trees, the animals, the sun, the soil, and the leaves.
- *Smell* the moist earth, the heavy scent of green vegetation.
- *Hear* the birds, sticks cracking, animals moving, creek flowing.
- *Feel* the cool moist air, the cool soil, the warm sun in a clearing.
- *Taste* the fresh water from a creek, a ripe berry, a sweet apple.
- *Be amazed* and in awe through your extrasensory perception.

Step 3. Enjoy Being in Your Pleasant Place.

Start off with 5 minutes then gradually expand your imagery time to about 15 - 20 minutes per day. Your skill with the visual-imagery-relaxation technique is built by repetition and concentration. Initially you may be distracted by internal bodily discomfort or external noises. With repeated use, you will become a master imagery wizard, able to concentrate with fewer distractions. You are building your mental muscles and preparing yourself for deeper visualization and mindfulness.

After you have become skilled at using the imagery relaxation technique, you can use parts of the technique in a shorter format (i.e., a few seconds or a few minutes) when you need a quick relaxation break.

My *Calm, Relaxed, & Free* meditation is available at my store: **store.duncantooley.com**

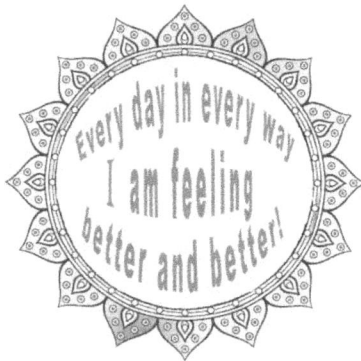

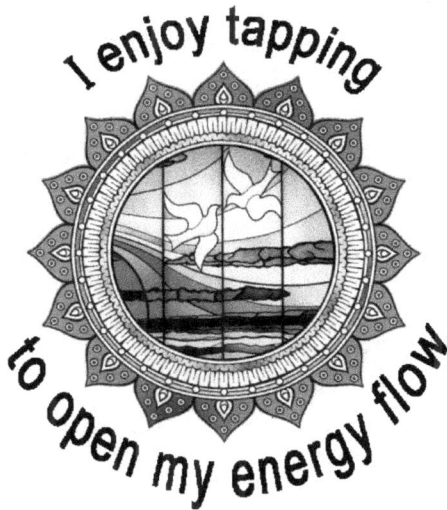

Chapter 5

I enjoy tapping

to open my energy flow

Acupressure

About Acupressure

Acupressure derives from acupuncture, a form of Chinese medicine that is thousands of years old. Acupuncture medicine is based on the belief that energy, called chi (say "chee"), flows through and around your body along pathways called meridians, and that illness is the result of blockages or imbalances in the flow. Needles are inserted at one or more access points (acupressure points) to improve the energy flow and relieve pain or illness. The needles are slightly larger than a hair, and hardly felt at all. Sometimes heat or electricity is added to the needles. Medical reviews conclude that acupuncture is effective for many types of pain. Acupressure is based on the same energy system as acupuncture and can be called *acupuncture without needles.*

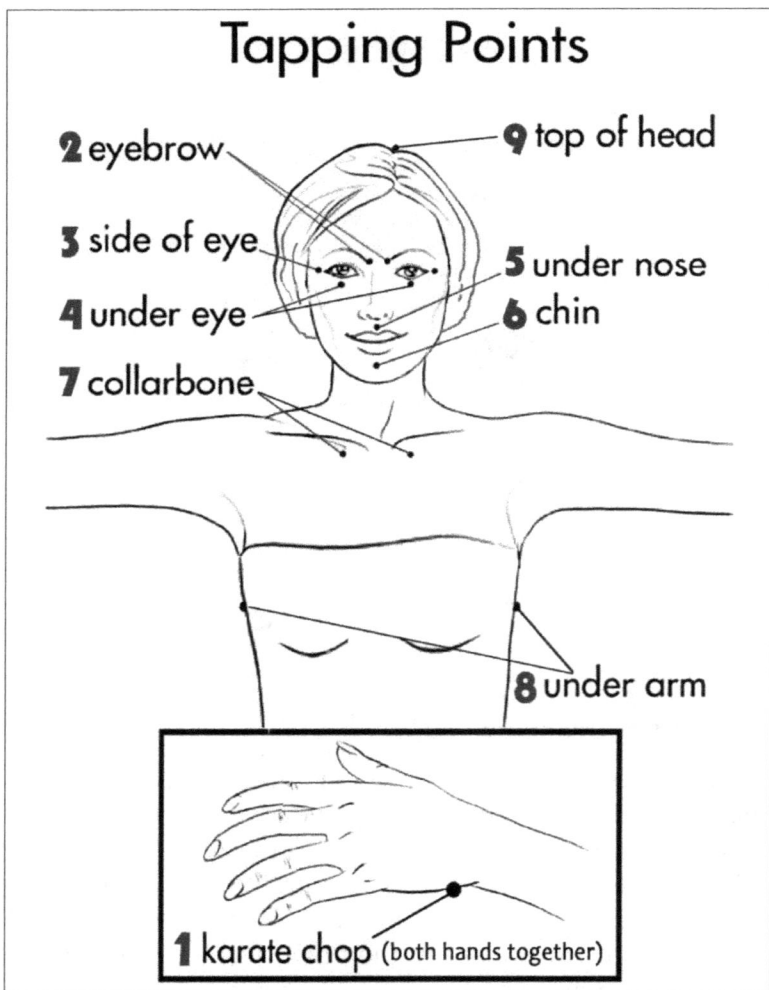

Tapping Points

2 eyebrow

9 top of head

3 side of eye

5 under nose

4 under eye

6 chin

7 collarbone

8 under arm

1 karate chop (both hands together)

Tapping on the acupressure points of the face and upper body while using specific language is a proven technique. Tapping for pain relief is a type of psychological acupuncture that effectively rewires the brain circuits and interrupts the pain cycle. Furthermore, tapping has a calming effect that relieves any stress or anxiety about the discomfort. Acupressure tapping is easy to learn to do it yourself without the assistance of another person.

Steps to Use Acupressure Point Tapping for Relief

Step 1. Prepare.
- Identify that area of your body where you are experiencing discomfort that you desire to change, and measure the intensity of the discomfort on a 1 to 10 scale.
- Construct *Phrase A:* "Even though I experience discomfort in my (name part of body from step 2)..."
- Construct *Phrase B:* "I choose to relax and feel great! I release whatever prevents me from being comfortable."
- Use the diagram for location of the 9 tapping points or symmetric point pairs.

Step 2. Tap on Your Hand.
- Say *Phrase A* aloud.
- Take a full breath in and say *Phrase B* on the exhale while tapping on tapping point #1 (side of hand).
- Repeat 2 more times (*Phrase A* without tapping, then *Phrase B* while tapping and exhaling).

Step 3. Tap on Points 2 through 9.
- Do the same process, (*Phrase A* no-tap; *Phrase B* exhaling & tapping), 3 times on each of the #2 through #9 tapping points (a total of 27 repetitions of *Phrases A & B*).
- Measure your comfort level at the end on a scale of 1 to 10 and notice the improvement. Repeat if desired.

Pro-Tip: *Tooley's Emotional Freedom Technique (TEFT):* The acupressure tapping process can also be used for creating happy emotions and habits when coupled with the appropriate phrases. This method differs from the traditional EFT in the wording of the phrases and the omission of tapping on the first phrase to prevent reinforcement of the undesired.

In *Phrase A,* state the trigger for the emotion or habit after the words *even though.* Example: "Even though I get really angry when my boss criticizes me."

Then formulate *Phrase B* as your new desired and chosen response beginning with the words *I choose.* Example: "I choose to be calm, relaxed, and at peace with myself."

Use the same process above. Measure the emotional intensity before and again afterward by recalling the experience with your eyes closed. It is OK if the words you say on each tap change; it is the evidence of the releasing of emotion (energy in motion). Notice how the emotion intensity is reduced.

Story: An older gentleman came to me to help relieve anxiety about being seen or heard using a public restroom. At work he had to cross the plant to use a remote restroom that was always vacant. He was unable to give a urine specimen at the doctor's office; he had to bring the jar home and then take it back to the doctor. In the army, he arose early to use the latrine before anyone else awoke. His anxiety about this topic had plagued him since adolescence.

Using my TEFT tapping process, his *Phrase A* was "Even though I am very anxious whenever I think of using a public restroom." His *Phrase B* was "I choose to be comfortable and relaxed and easily do so."

During the process, his *Phrase A* spontaneously changed to "Even though my mother taught me that using the toilet was dirty." Afterward he explained that his family moved to a new house when he was a teenager. After any guest came to their house, his mother would immediately go clean the toilet. The lesson he subconsciously took from his mother's habit had plagued him his whole life!

When I called him the next day, he confirmed that he had easily used the active restroom across the hall from his office.

Extra: The diagram of tapping points with procedure on a single sheet is available for printing at the book extras website: *www.feelgreat.duncantooley.com*

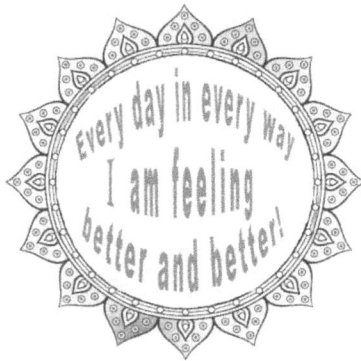

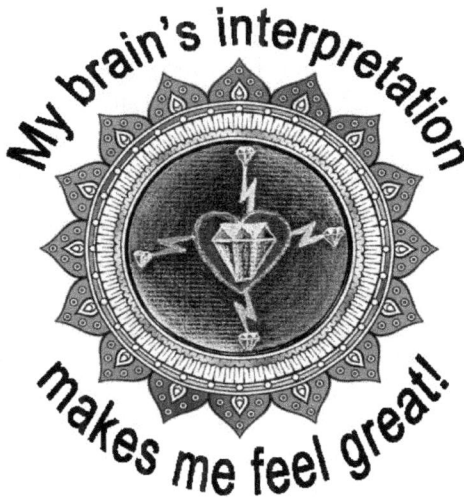

Chapter 6

TENS

About TENS

TENS is the abbreviation for *Transcutaneous Electrical Nerve Stimulator.* TENS is a device that can block pain by electrical stimulations on the skin at or surrounding the point of pain. Although there are different types of TENS units, the one described below is the portable one that worked for me to relieve the residual nuisance pain from a vertebrae disc rupture.

The TENS is a small electrical oscillator about the size of a thick cell phone that produces an electrical wave form and sends that wave to dual channels of outputs. The wave shape and oscillation frequency can be adjusted, providing a wide spectrum of pulse patterns that can be delivered to your body. Each channel has two electrode pads that attach to the skin. A continuous electrical pulse waveform is sent between the electrodes, causing a sensation of electrical shock. The intensity is adjusted to just below the maximum tolerable level.

> *My Story:* One day in 1986 I lifted too many heavy doors. The next morning, I was surprised to find that I had wet the bed. As I stepped out of bed, I crashed to the floor because of intense pain in my right thigh. Later I learned that a disc between two of my lower vertebrae ruptured during the night, probably strained though lifting all those doors. That was the beginning of my back pain saga!
>
> I had back surgery (discectomy) to clean up the disc debris and remove the pressure on the leg nerve. The surgeon said that I would probably see him again. He was right! After recovering from the initial surgery, I had a different vertebrae disc rupture several years later. Again I had the back surgery that remedied the pain in my other leg.
>
> When I had a third back incident several years later, I said "No more surgery; show me a rehabilitation doctor instead of a surgeon." The rehabilitation doctor prescribed a TENS unit for me and arranged for a physical therapist to show me how to use it.
>
> My first TENS experience was not good! I followed the instructions to use it for no more than 20 minutes at a time, as often as every hour. Its use had the effect of increasing the intensity of the pain instead of reducing it. I went back to the physical therapist the next day. The therapist made some adjustments to the

controls inside that vary the wave form and frequency and instructed me to use it again.

I placed the electrode pairs above and below the problem vertebra, clipped the TENS oscillator on my belt and adjusted the intensity controls to feel a sharp kick. I then went about my regular work and forgot about it. About 15 minutes later I noticed that the lights on the TENS were still illuminated. I felt nothing, no pain, and no electrical stimulation. I turned the unit off, leaving the electrodes in place.

Later when the pain returned, I switched the TENS on and adjusted the intensity. A short time later, I experienced the same surprise at finding the lights still on and feeling no stimulation or pain. That first day I used the TENS eight times. The next day I used it six times. Over the next week, as my pain decreased, so did my use of the TENS. After the second week, my early morning pain was removed by use of the TENS once in the morning, and I remained comfortable all day.

Soon my frequency of use dropped to about once per week. Within a couple of months my discomfort became so infrequent that I only used the TENS about once a month. Eventually a year passed without its use. Now I haven't used my TENS in the last 10 years.

What I notice is that I NEVER get back or leg discomfort, no matter what I do that might have previously caused pain. I believe the TENS has trained my brain into a habit of ignoring any nuisance back discomfort, even if I do some activity that would ordinarily have caused it.

How does TENS work?

My experience of the TENS seemed to work by fatiguing the attention my brain required to distinguish between the TENS pain (electrical shock) and the pinched nerve pain from the disc rupture. It was as if my brain got tired of identifying which stimulation was from the TENS and which was the real pain, so it gave up trying and switched both off!

The scientific explanation of a TENS operation is based on the *Gate Control Theory* of how pain is transmitted. The gate theory states that the nerves responding to touch, pressure, and vibration send their signals more rapidly and slam the gate closed behind them to the slower-moving signals of the pain neurons. Therefore, flooding the sensory system with touch, pressure, or vibration blocks pain. The electrical stimulation of the TENS triggers touch and vibration neurons that race ahead to the brain and block the signal from the pain neurons. A second theory hypothesizes that the electrical pulses stimulate the body to release its own pain-killing molecules, called endorphins, into the fluid bathing the spinal cord.

These explanations only cover the blocking of pain while the TENS is being used. What I experienced was the building of a *habit* of blocking the experience of pain. That habit trained my brain to ignore back pain whenever and whatever the cause, confirming that you can train your brain to end the pain and feel great!

Options to Use a TENS for Relief

Option A. Explore TENS Availability.
Inquire about TENS therapy in a conversation with your health care provider. This may get you a TENS unit at low or no cost that is properly set by a physical therapist.

Option B. Use a Mini-TENS.
Acquire one of the new simplified mini-TENS units available over-the-counter that has preset programs you can select. These appear to be a very practical and affordable solution for putting an end to nuisance pain.

Like all the other techniques in this book, they use the power of the brain to switch off the pain!

Option C. Purchase a Professional TENS

A professional TENS like I used has a wide range of settings available. Experiment with adjusting the settings yourself, or take to a professional for help with the initial settings

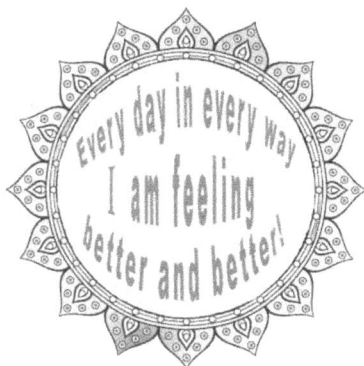

Every day in every way I am feeling better and better!

.

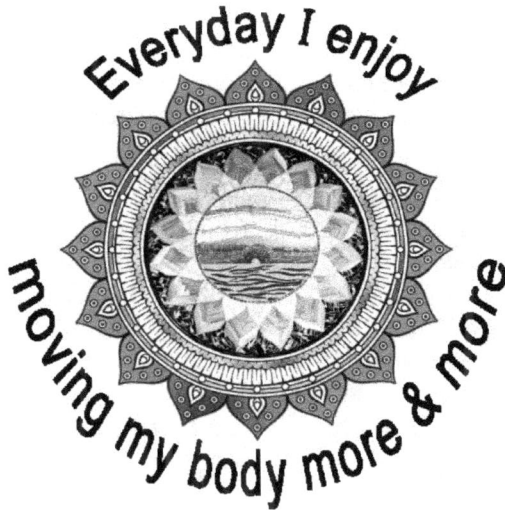

Chapter 7

Physical Exercise

About Physical Exercise

Studies show that physical exercise lowers pain thresholds. Practically speaking, what this means is that any physical condition in your body feels more comfortable when your flexibility and muscle tone are maintained by regular exercise.

The old prescription of bed rest for chronic back pain is no longer the recommendation. Now motion to lubricate

65

joints is the popular solution. A good fitness coach or exercise program works wonders.

> **Study:** *"Vigorous exercise has been shown to lead to significant alterations in the body's intrinsic pain-regulatory system. It can lead to increased serum levels of beta-endorphins, which are hundreds of times more powerful than the equivalent dose of morphine."* (Cf. References, Study 2)

> **Pro-Tip:** Select some suitable affirmations and repeat them during your exercise. Repetition of affirmations or mantras during physical exercise provides a more complete body-mind tuning for relief. This is similar to the way the physical poses of yoga complement the mind-focusing aspects of yoga.

Steps to Use Physical Exercise for Relief

Step 1. Choose Your Type of Exercise.

Physical therapy from a trained practitioner is an excellent means of relief. If regular physical therapy is not available, get instruction for home exercises. Get a home exercise DVD program or piece of equipment. Go to the gym. Do wall pushups while you heat your coffee or tea. Walking is an excellent exercise that is even better when done rapidly and with intention and focus. It can be a "meditation in motion."

Step 2. Make a Plan.

Put your exercise time into your daily calendar with reminders. Whatever you decide, make a plan! Decide how you will incorporate mindfulness, affirmations, and mantras into your program.

Step 3. Follow your plan.

Do the activity that you put in your plan. On schedule-challenged days, at least walk around the block. Walk your dog. Walk around a loop in your house if you can't get out! Just make daily exercise part of your comfort solution. You will feel better and better.

Step 4. Make Yourself Accountable.

Have a checklist or log to keep yourself accountable. Exercise with a group and commit that you will show up. Check-in daily with a like-minded accountability partner.

Step 5. Boost Your Motivation.

What if you really don't enjoy exercise and find sticking to a plan a challenge? Give your motivation a boost by adding a social or emotional element to it. Go with a friend or join a group that exercises together regularly. Any method that puts more fun in the experience will help you stick with it.

Hypnosis has helped change beliefs about the enjoyment and desirability of exercise with some of my clients and stimulated them to exercise more and enjoy it more. *More Fun Exercise* is a purposeful hypnotic meditation that stimulates your sub-conscience to desire more exercise. It is available at ***store.duncantooley.com***

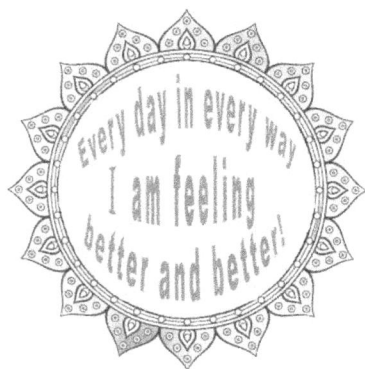

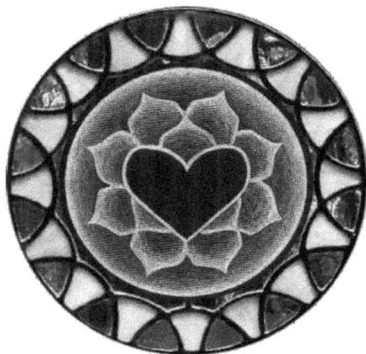

MIND-BASED METHODS
TO FEEL GREAT AGAIN

▶ **8. Tune Your Mindset**

▶ **9. Positive Self-Talk**

▶ **10. Visualization**

▶ **11. Affirmation-Afformation**

▶ **12. Control Center**

▶ **13. Hypnosis**

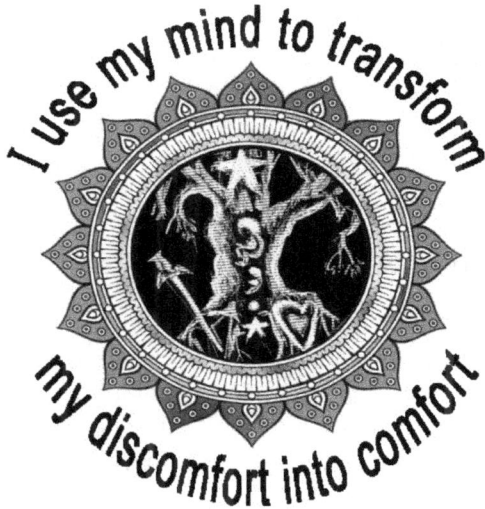

Chapter 8

I use my mind to transform my discomfort into comfort

Tune Your Mindset

"First and foremost, attack the pain where you can do the most good—in your mind."-- Peter G. Lehndorff

About Mindset

What you believe about pain and your relationship to pain is the most important single factor in how you feel and to what extent you suffer, if any. Tuning your mindset is the technique of changing your beliefs about pain and how you will react to it. Begin training your brain to feel great again by fully applying this brain re-programming technique.

> *"Pain and suffering are different things. Pain is a physical sensation. Suffering is one possible reaction to that sensation. But suffering is not the only possible reaction to pain. It's possible to experience pain without suffering from it. When you learn to experience pain without suffering, you will be set free. You will be able to love your life again, even though your life may still contain some pain, as all lives do."* --Dharma Singh Khalsa

Steps to Tune Your Mindset for Relief

Step 1. Decide to Take Control.

You are not your pain! It is not you! You don't have to own it! When you take charge of how you feel, you give up feeling like you are doomed to suffer. The first step to tuning your mindset is your decision to take control. This converts you from victim to victor! Decide right now that pain is powerless and that you are in total control of how you feel!

Step 2. Make a Proclamation.

Say this proclamation aloud 10 times, letting its truth sink deeper and deeper into every neuron of your brain and every cell of your body:

> **"I am in charge of my mind and now transform discomfort into comfort."**

Congratulations! Now that you have decided to take control, you are already past the hardest part. You have tuned your mind to be successful, and it will be so because your mind is in control!

Step 3. Set the Goal for Your Feel Great Life.

What will your life be like once pain is gone and you feel great? This is the goal that makes you smile. It is your *Feel Great* life you enjoy and desire to have again.

Will you have greater range of motion and more flexibility? Will you dance, play golf or tennis, sew, bicycle ride? What goal are you setting for yourself when all discomfort is past history and you feel great? What will you be doing and feeling? Imagine that future as if it is real now.

Make a proclamation of your goal for your *Feel Great* life. (State it as if you are experiencing it already).

Some examples are:

- *"I enjoy playing tennis with my friends twice a week."*
- *"I love walking my dog 2 miles every day."*
- *"I enjoy dancing (yoga, bicycling, swimming) again."*
- *"I love having my old (great) life back again!"*

Write your goal proclamation here: "I (am) _____ _____."

Say your goal proclamation aloud 10 times. Each time you say it, let its truth sink a little deeper into every neuron of your brain and every cell of your body.

Step 4. Set Your Comfort Level.

Now that you have clarified your goal of what your life will be like, it is time to set your comfort level. How much do you want discomfort to diminish? By when?

Make a proclamation about your Comfort Level. (State it as if it is "already becoming" the level you desire).

Some examples are:

- *"My comfort level continues to increase 20% each week."*
- *"I am feeling better each day as I use my favorite comfort-building technique (from this book) every day."*
- *"By the end of next week I will be totally comfortable doing* (your choice of activity*)."*

Write your comfort level proclamation here:

"_____"

Say your comfort level proclamation aloud 10 times. Each time you say it, let its truth sink a little deeper into every neuron of your brain and every cell of your body.

Step 5. Set Your Investment and Measurement.

"What is not measured is not achieved." — *Japanese proverb*

- How much time and energy will you invest in finding your best technique(s) to banish discomfort?
  _____

- How will you track your progress? _____
  _____

- What time of day will you devote each day to your comfort transformation? _____

- Do you have your journal to keep track of any discomfort and the technique(s) that you are using? _____ If not, get one!

Step 6. Congratulate Yourself!

You have tuned your mindset for success at feeling great quickly. You are already well underway to achieving what you desire! You are training your brain! You have taken the essential steps to tune your mind for the changes you desire.

> **Extra:** Download and print a *Tune Your Mindset* worksheet so you can keep your written answers for easy reference: *www.feelgreat.duncantooley.com*

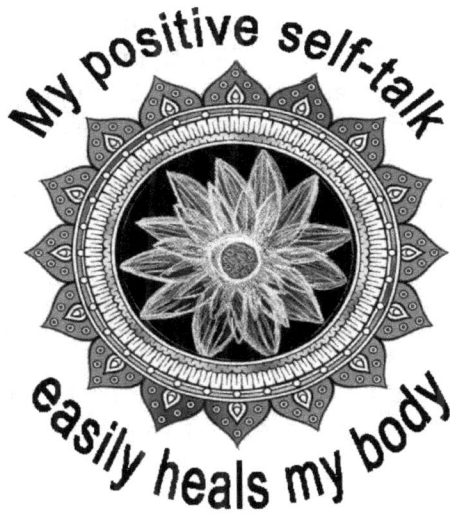

Chapter 9

My positive self-talk easily heals my body

Positive Self-Talk

About Positive Self-Talk

This technique diminishes discomfort by changing your vocabulary in your self-talk, and subsequently in your external speech, about how you feel. Language plays a powerful role in how you feel. Every cell of your body communicates with other cells. The messages flowing through billions of neurons in your brain affect every part of your body. You absorb pain information from TV, from your family, from your doctor, and especially from your own self-talk. It all affects how you feel.

With the Positive Self-Talk technique, you take control of the language you permit to enter your mind and body. You become the gatekeeper rather than a sponge absorbing negative language and letting that language affect you. When you decide to implement monitoring your self-talk and keeping it always positive, you are committing to a life-changing plan of action that takes vigilance, determination, and courage, at first.

Like everything you do in life, the process becomes easier with repetition. When repeated often enough, the process eventually slips down into your subconscious where it becomes an automatic habit without thought. Keeping your self-talk positive is one of the most powerful long-term habits to develop.

Self-Talk Starts Early

When you were a child and you were learning to do something, perhaps learn a new task, you probably spoke instructions aloud to yourself to get it right. Maybe when learning to tie your shoes, you repeated "left over right, then tuck under..." or something like that. Maybe you repeated your home telephone number aloud as you walked to school so you would remember it if needed. As you grew older, you internalized this conversation to become your self-talk. You also incorporated the instructions, commands, and scoldings of your parents, teachers, and other significant authority figures, including doctors and religious ministers. You added what your friends called you. This voice that chatters all the time in your head is the composite voice of all that you have absorbed and believe about yourself, and which perpetuates the status-quo as your ego control task-master.

More than Words

But self-talk is not only the words that you internally "speak" to yourself (normally in your native tongue), but also the promptings from your sub-conscious that may surface as impulses rather than words.

Examples of self-talk that are conscious and words:

- I glance at the clock and tell myself, "I still have 45 minutes before I have to leave."
- I see the dishes piled in the kitchen sink and say to myself, "What a mess; you need to wash these!"
- "I've got to get to sleep! I've got to get to sleep! I've got to get to sleep!"

Examples of self-talk that are sub-conscious and automatic:

- My urge to grab for a cookie each time I walk into the kitchen where the full cookie jar is in unobstructed view.
- My "Stupid!" when I stub my toe on the chair leg.
- My "I can't; I'm not good enough" when I have a thought about a magnificent idea I want to pursue.

This voice in your head is a universal thing. We all have one. Scientists say that we have about 60,000 thoughts every day and that most of these are the same as yesterday. It's those thoughts that constitute self-talk either in a default auto-mode or a deliberate choice mode.

Self-talk affects what we believe and what we do. We can use self-talk deliberately to guide us through difficult or complex situations. Sometimes we create an instruction list for ourselves that becomes our self-talk.

Self-talk affects our emotional state. Deliberately choosing to flow a stream of "up" self-dialogue when you are feeling "down" is an effective, quick, and inexpensive picker-upper!

My Story: I notice my self-talk and hear these instructions:

- Every time I exit my front door, *"Check: Do I have wallet, keys, and cell phone?"*
- When confronted with an "I-E-specific" spelling challenge, *"I before E, except after C, or when it sounds like 'A' as in 'neighbor' and 'weigh.'"*

Self-Talk Studies

The effects of self-talk have been widely studied and documented in the field of sports. As a result, a key component of all athletic coaching is training in self-talk for a positive and successful outcome. Is there any reason to believe that the results of self-talk are any different for the rest of us non-athletes? Of course not! It is clear that self-talk affects what we do, how we feel, and what our life is like!

A popular type of therapy, Cognitive Behavior Therapy (CBT), is based on repairing poor self-talk. The concept is that erroneous, distorted thoughts contribute to painful mood states such as anxiety or depression. The corrective practice is to keep a log of one's negative statements about oneself (your self-talk) and replace them with more positive and adaptive ones. Research supports the effectiveness of such measures and the resultant restructured thought and behavior patterns. (Hypnosis is much quicker and more efficient at achieving even better results. See the comparative study cited in *Appendix A7, Hypnosis Myths Busted*, Myth 10.)

Monitoring your self-talk and noticing when it is positive or negative is a very worthwhile discipline because you are auto-programming yourself with your daily self-talk. The path to lasting change employs a monitored and well-nourished self-talk.

Words Affect You

Words are not sterile, pristine things! They affect you because of all that you have stored deep within your psyche. The meaning of every word in your vocabulary is a compilation of what you absorbed through your social history. That means that every word is flavored (contaminated, infected) with the meanings and emotions of your parents, educators, and heroes, and your past experiences.

This applies to *PAIN* and all its word relatives (like hurt, ache, throb, sting, suffer, agony, distress, etc.). Just the thought of the word *PAIN* fires thousands of your brain's neurons to bring forth all the past associations. This is just the normal way your brain works, bringing up all the connections with each word.

Why is this important?

Your understanding of the power of language, the power of specific words, puts you in control of triggering (or not) all the memories and emotions that are associated with specific words. What if you could disconnect from all the history, emotions, and discomfort associated with PAIN? It's easy; one of the powerful techniques for feeling great and reducing your discomfort is to change the language you use.

Your choice of words matters.
Your life depends on it!

Steps to Use Positive Self-Talk for Relief

Step 1. Banish the Word "PAIN" from Your Vocabulary.

Decide that in the future, "PAIN" is one of those vulgar and forbidden 4-letter words. Instead, talk only about your "comfort level." Your comfort level may be higher or lower at certain times, but you never experience that P@#$ word! Your comfort level may not be as high as you desire on days when the source of your discomfort is acting up.

Step 2. Create Your "Self-Talk Monitor."

Dedicate a small portion of your brain to objectively monitor your self-talk. Its job is to monitor all the self-talk and thoughts similar to the way hall monitors watch high school students to make sure they follow the school rules. Your Self-Talk Monitor listens to each self-talk expression and peeks at every thought that comes floating through your mind. Your Self-Talk Monitor examines these thoughts to ensure that they are positive in outlook and do not contain any references to P@#$.

If the P@#$ word (or any of its nasty cousins) shows up, or if your self-talk is negative in any way, your Self Talk Monitor immediately says "Cancel! Cancel! Out of here!" and substitutes instead a positive replacement.

Undesired thoughts can be frequent and persistent. Be patient and encouraging with yourself as you accept the challenge to filter out negativity as these thoughts attempt to pass through your mind. With practice at monitoring your thoughts and words, you will learn to interrupt, cancel, and replace negativity. Your decision to avoid/replace them and your monitoring efforts will cause the negative thoughts to present themselves less and less frequently.

Step 3. Banish the Word P@#$ from Your Environment.

Request your friends and family not to speak to you using that P@#$ word. Inform them that you no longer have any of the P@#$ stuff; you only have a comfort level now. Switch off TV news or commercials about P@#$, especially the pharmaceutical company advertisements.

Step 4. Engage Powerful Positive Thoughts.

Develop some thoughts that reinforce the end of your discomfort and say them often, especially if a negative thought appears. Here are some examples:

- *"My comfort level is increasing more and more each day."*
- *"My happy mind controls my healthy body."*
- *"I am grateful for my health and happiness."*
- *"I feel GREAT today!"*

The more frequently you say these phrases, internally and out loud, the more you radiate the positive energy that makes the statements 100% reality. More information about constructing positive statements is found in Chapter 11, *Affirmations.*

> ***Pro-tip:*** The power of language goes way beyond your sensation and interpretation of discomfort. Language literally affects everything in your life. The words that you use to express every feeling to yourself flavor your current experience with the automatic input from your database of past experiences associated with that language. Master the use of better-feeling language about your comfort level, and then apply these rules to every area of your life. Use words that you associate with the most pleasant emotions when you speak to yourself, and your life will become much more joyful!

> ***Extra:*** Get the list of powerful Positive Words from the book extras website: *www.feelgreat.duncantooley.com.* Use them to replace negative words in your self-talk. Use them later to formulate your affirmations

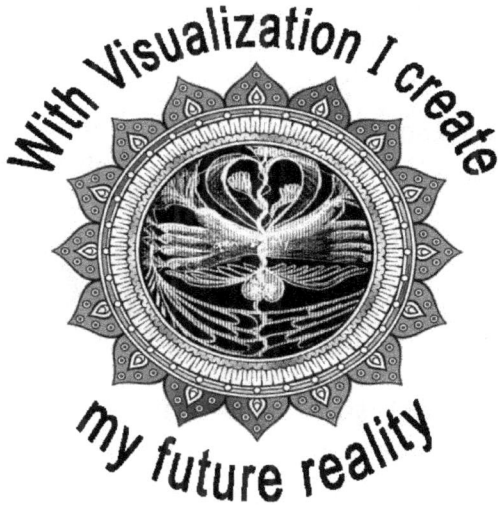

Chapter 10

With Visualization I create my future reality

Visualization

"Whenever you play healing images through your mind, a healing process takes place, even if you are not consciously aware of it--and even if you do not completely believe it will work." --Norman J. Marcus

About Visualization

This technique is built upon the power and importance of your imagination. Information and instructions from your imagination are accepted and processed by your subconscious equally to the way it accepts information and instructions from your memory and your senses. The technique gives your subconscious mind a story, a very sensory story in vivid detail! In your story you feel wonderful and enjoy yourself. You are fascinated with life and having fun. Your enjoyable story captures your attention, energizes you, and releases endorphins that cause you to feel good.

Visualization is sometimes called *Guided Imagery* because you guide your mind to imagine details of a specific scenario or story. You call upon all of your senses to create the "imagery" and you are the "guide." Visualization builds upon and extends your imagery skill from Chapter 4, *Relaxation Response,* by adding details of a story or scenario for your subconscious to create a specific result.

Options to Use Visualization (or Guided Imagery)

There are several options to use Visualization or Guided Imagery for relief:

Option A. Guided Meditation Event Method

Steps to Use the Event Method for Relief

Step 1. Find a Suitable Event.

A guided meditation event is perhaps the easiest way to start because the visualization structure is provided by someone else. All you have to do then is relax and follow along with your imagination. There are workshops, classes, or groups where the guided meditation (visualization) is led by an instructor or facilitator. Search out several and select the one that seems most appropriate for what you desire.

Step 2. Participate.

You fill in all the details and sensory experiences that are only hinted by the meditation leader. Personalize the general instructions to make the experience uniquely

84

yours. Include what you want for your outcome, even if the leader fails to invite you to experience it.

Step 3. Remember (or Record) the Visualization.

Learn from the imagery and commands, and then you can create your own more personalized visualization for yourself as described later.

~ ◻ ~ ◻ ~ ◻ ~

Option B. Recorded Visualization Method

Steps to Use a Recorded Visualization for Relief

A recorded guided visualization offers all of the advantages of a meditation event in the comfort of your home (or wherever else you choose). Audio and video files now play back on cell phones, computers, TV's, and other devices.

Step 1. Acquire a Suitable Recorded Visualization.

Each of my recorded guided meditations (visualizations) is carefully crafted for their specific purpose. Go to *store.DuncanTooley.com* for information about my recorded visualizations.

Step 2. Use the Visualization to Meditate.

You just close your eyes, drift off, relax, follow the guidance instructions and soon you are feeling wonderful!

Step 3. Use As a Model to Create Your Own.

Remember the structure of the visualization. See the options below for creating your own personalized guided meditations.

~ ◻ ~ ◻ ~ ◻ ~

Option C. Spontaneous Method

Steps to Use Spontaneous Visualization for Relief

Step 1. Plan and Prepare.

- Set your intention for what you want the effect of this particular visualization experience to be.
- Decide where you want to go to relax (what your private sanctuary will be like).
- Formulate what you want to happen there.

Step 2. Begin Your Journey.

- Relax; close your eyes; play soft music (optional); take some deep breaths.
- Begin to imagine yourself on your journey and notice everything: the colors, the scenery, the aromas, your feelings, the sounds, the tastes, anything else that strikes you as pleasant or extraordinary. Let your imagination have a wonderful daydream.

Step 3. Enjoy Your Sanctuary.

- Arrive at your sanctuary and enjoy it. Notice everything about it, every sensual aspect, so that you can return there in the future.
- Let whatever you wanted to happen in your sanctuary unfold. Imagine achieving all of your goals, finding the relationships that you desire, and being fantastically happy, or whatever else you desire.
- Bask in the satisfying glow of the feeling of being completely fulfilled and happy. Decide what you will bring back with you when you leave your sanctuary.

Step 4. Return.

- Leave your sanctuary and backtrack on the path you took to get there (or optionally, take another interesting way back).
- Be clear about what you are bringing back with you and carry it carefully.

- Come back from your visualization by giving yourself three instructions:
  - ○ Become aware of your external surroundings.
  - ○ Move your feet, legs, hands, arms, and head.
  - ○ Open your eyes feeling re-energized and refreshed.

~□~□~□~

Option D. Personal Recorded Method.

Steps to Use Personal Recorded Visualization for Relief

Step 1. Prepare.

- Decide where you want to go to relax (your private sanctuary) and what you want to happen while you are there.
- Write a script as if you were giving someone commands about how to journey through the visualization. Your script will become the recorded voice of the "guide" who will lead you through your guided visualization.
- Get your recording device ready and practice with it.

Step 2. Record the script as your own guide.

- Address yourself by name.
- Speak very slowly to give yourself time to hear the commands and then to carry them out.
- You could have some soft music playing while you are recording. If you or someone you know has the skill, add a music track to your recording later.

Step 3. Meditate.

- Get comfortable, relax, take some deep breaths, start your recording playback, and close your eyes.
- Follow your guided visualization through to its end.

- If you did not record coming back at the end, give yourself the three instructions to come back as in the last step of Option C, Spontaneous Method.

Step 4. Evaluate Your Visualization.

- How well did your visualization script work for you?
- Where there any things omitted or not clear?
- Are you getting the result you intended?
- Should you change something in the recording? If so, do it before your next use.

Pro-Tip: Make your own recorded guided meditations using the free download audio program *Audacity,* which includes these features important for recording and editing your script:

1) *Record directly from your laptop or tablet microphone*
2) *Import a recording made on your phone (or anywhere)*
3) *Easily make corrections with highlight-cut-paste editing*
4) *Add music by adding and mixing multiple tracks*
5) *Control and balance the volume on multiple tracks*
6) *Output as audio mp3 file for replay on a variety of devices*

Chapter 11

My affirmations confirm my coming experiences

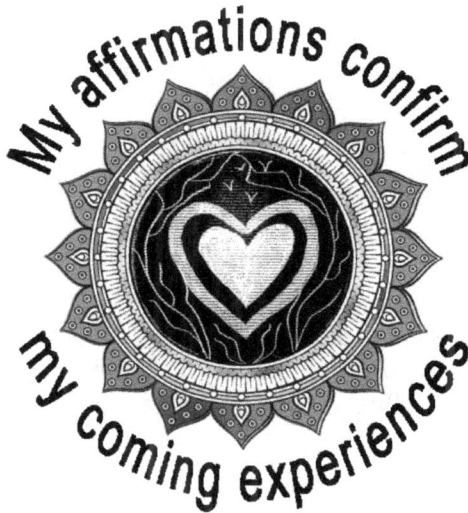

Affirmation - Afformation

About Affirmations

Affirmations are short messages to your subconscious for the purpose of strengthening a belief and prompting your subconscious to act in alignment with that belief. They are instructions to yourself about what you desire to believe to be true. The instruction has the effect of becoming absolutely true in every sense such that you *know* and *experience* its truth.

The goal of using affirmations is to move from *desiring* to *believing*, to *knowing with absolute certainty*, the truth stated in the affirmation. The goal is that there is not the slightest doubt about the validity of that truth. That certainty, absence of even the smallest doubt, is what guarantees your affirmation is already becoming reality!

Belief vs. Certainty

The power of affirmations is in the difference between belief and certainty. I once considered myself a very religious person and thought that my strong belief was the highest form of faith. Then I learned that belief is not enough! There is a tiny *lie* hidden in be*lie*f, a small doubt that can hold you back from complete certainty. The difference is illustrated by the following thought experiment:

Imagine holding a book out at arm's length and ask yourself "What will happen when I release it?" You won't say "I BELIEVE the book will hit the floor." I predict you will say something like: "The book will hit the floor."

And if questioned about your certainty of that result, you would say something like, "I KNOW it will hit the floor. I am certain it will hit the floor. I have not the slightest doubt that it will hit the floor."

The book falls because it obeys the Law of Gravity, which states: "Objects with physical mass attract each other." The earth pulls on a book with the same force that the book pulls on the earth. The book moves more toward the earth because its small mass moves more easily than the much larger mass of the earth. The force of attraction is the same however.

Every particle in the universe attracts every other particle. Water molecules attract the moon as strongly as the moon attracts the ocean's water molecules. The water molecules move upward and result in high tides without moving the moon out of its orbit.

Law of Attraction

The Law of Gravity is a subset of the general Law of Attraction. The attraction effect applies not just to objects with mass, but to all things. The Law applies to people being attracted to each other, to circumstances, to emotions, and to events. And, yes, the Law even applies to P@#$ (See Positive Self-Talk steps). Your thoughts attract more thoughts of comfort or discomfort, whichever you choose!

Some proverbs you may already know summarize the Law of Attraction's effects:

- *"Birds of a feather flock together."*

- *"What goes around comes around."*

- *"What you think about, comes about!"*

- *"What you think about (believe & tell yourself) is what you get (is attracted to you). "*

The Law of Attraction is always working whether we acknowledge the Law or not. Affirmations work with the Law of Attraction to get the relief we desire.

Steps to Use Affirmations for Relief
Step 1. Compose Your Affirmations.

- Use short, simple, easily repeatable declarative sentences.
- Use the present tense (no futures or potentials).
- Use only positive words (no form of negatives).

- Use only words of things you desire (no mention of things you don't want; for example, instead of "I am pain-free," use "I feel great!").
- Make your affirmation about you (not about other people, events, circumstances, or things).
- Use strong, emotional words, with *juice* or power (*beautiful, fantastic, awesome,* and *magnificent* are more powerful than *good*).
- Conclude with: "I am grateful that this or something better, is manifesting for me right now!"

Step 2. Use Proven Relief & Comfort Affirmations.

Affirmations that end discomfort and increase comfort and well-being that have proven their value with clients over the years are listed below. Most were gleaned from the writings of Shelley Stockwell-Nicholas, PhD.

- I feel GREAT!
- My life is a celebration.
- Everything I do allows me to enjoy my life more and more.
- I am healthy.
- My positive thoughts create my healthy body.
- My body is my perfect friend. I take care of my body.
- I am fully in tune with my body.
- I exercise and eat only healthy foods.
- I control my body with my mind.
- I have within me a creative force that knows how to repair my body, restore every cell to perfect health, and regenerate lost cells. I am grateful that it is working within me every minute of every day.

- I give myself to my highest power. I give myself to that part of me that knows exactly what I need to do to be happy, comfortable, and radiant.
- I give my body the "OK" to heal itself.
- I command my body to repair and renew itself now!
- I forgive myself for any mistakes I have made.
- In this moment I am cleansed.
- I learn from the past and then let the past go.
- I am joy.
- In this NOW moment I am happy, comfortable and radiant.
- I know my body can heal itself. I command my body to heal itself now.
- As I breathe, every nerve, ligament, muscle, bone, fiber, and organ of my body comes into balance.
- The creative force within me heals me and keeps me well!
- All my body functions work perfectly and I know it!
- I feel terrific!
- Every little cell in my body is *happy* and *well*!"

Step 3. Make the Affirmations Part of Your Daily Life.

- Say them often. Write them. Post them where you see them. Chant them.
- Record them with feeling and listen to your recording often.
- Say or play them as you fall asleep at night and first thing upon awakening.
- Trust, allow, accept, believe, and *know* that they are already working for you!

Step 4. Repeat, Repeat, Repeat.

In 1932 Aldous Huxley wrote in *Brave New World,* "62,400 repetitions make one truth!" That number may be an exaggeration, but the *repetition truth effect,* has been verified in many scientific studies.

> ***Study:*** After examining fifty-one studies since 1977 on the repetition truth effect, the researchers concluded that the more we are exposed to a statement, the more likely we are to come to believe that it is true. (Cf. References, Study 3)

Confirmation of this study is easily seen in the billions of dollars spent in advertising based on merely repeatedly telling consumers that "our product is superior to others" will sooner or later lead them to believe it to be true, and finally to purchase that product instead of a competitor's.

Sports psychologists have clearly shown that an athlete's performance can be diminished if the athlete has the habit of repeating, thinking, and saying negative statements about herself and her performance. Likewise, performance is improved if the athlete has a habit of repeating positive statements about self, success, and accomplishment.

> ***Pro-Tip:*** Determine your favorite affirmations and write them on six index cards. Place one card on your vanity mirror, refrigerator, car dashboard, computer monitor, night table, and in your wallet or purse. Say your affirmations from the card every time you see it. The one on your night table is the reminder to say your affirmations as you fall asleep and first thing upon awakening because these are the two most powerful times to do so.

> ***Extra:*** Get a great list of affirmations at the book extras site: *www.feelgreat.duncantooley.com.*

~ ¤ ~ ¤ ~ ¤ ~

About Afformations

Afformations are included in this chapter because, like affirmations, they focus on the positive. The key difference, however, is the afformation asks a positive question rather than making a statement.

An afformation takes the statement of positive condition from an affirmation and turns it into a question based on the positive condition having already happened. Afformations turn the positive truth into a question based on Noah St. John's book, *The Secret Code of Success.* Rather than just stating something is true (as with an affirmation), an afformation asks *why* it is true. For being comfortable and feeling great today, your afformation might ask, "Why do I feel great today?" or ""How is it so easy for my thoughts to make me feel great?"

According to St. John, our minds appreciate questions and are eager to search for answers. He likens this process to an *automatic search function* in the brain. He maintains that afformations remain stimulating and challenging over time independent of the power of repeated affirmations over time.

Steps to Use Afformations for Relief

Step 1. Begin with Your Affirmations.

Create your affirmations using the process above to state the change that you desire as affirmed and already done.

Step 2. Create Your Afformation.

Formulate a question that acknowledges you already have what you want. For example, if you want to be healthy, ask "Why am I healthy?" or "What is happening in my body to cause my good health?" or "How did I get so healthy?" The question triggers the auto search function in your brain.

Step 3. Notice the Answers to Your Question.

Most likely your mind will present positive potential answers to the puzzle question. More answers will continue to flow. These thoughts may lead to even more questions and positive thoughts. Keep going! They will reinforce your great feeling as each potential answer your brain offers will reinforce your certainty of it becoming your actual condition.

Step 4. Make Afformation Questions a Habit.

Each week formulate a new afformation question on a different aspect or goal. You will attract what you seek based on your thoughts and positive vibrations. You will notice the change in thinking, actions, and feelings that follows from regular use of afformations.

> ***Pro-tip:*** Create for yourself a mix of affirmations and afformations, with several affirmations to each afformation that asks why the affirmations are working. If you followed the Pro-Tip for affirmations above, add an afformation on your index cards.

Chapter 12

I easily turn up my comfort control to high

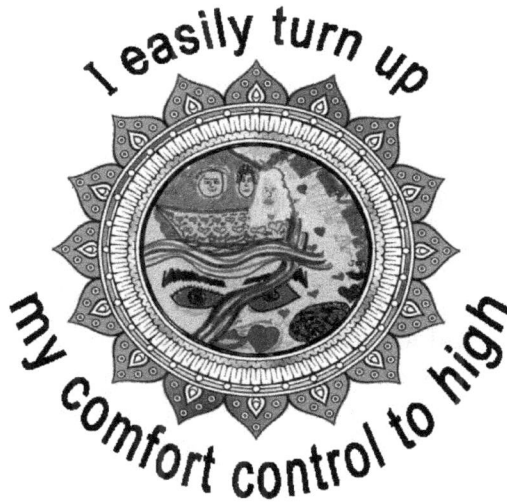

Control Center

About Control Center

The Control Center technique works on a very familiar concept and yet is extremely powerful. The technique is easily applied because of your familiarity and experience with a common household control, the thermostat.

The industrial control center is the brains and heart of modern manufacturing and service industries. Movies show images of the control centers for power plants and manufacturing complexes. Advertisements show the control dispatch centers for emergency services. The dashboard in your car is a kind of mini control center for the functions of your vehicle.

The fundamental process behind every control in a control center is the *monitor-and-adjust feedback loop* composed of 4 steps:

1. Set the desired set-point (control point)
2. Measure performance against the set-point
3. Take corrective action if necessary
4. Loop back to Step 2.

A simple example of a monitor-and-adjust control is the thermostat in your home or car. If you set the thermostat for 70 degrees (Fahrenheit), and the air conditioner and heater are operative, then your temperature will remain in a tight range (usually about ±½ degree) around 70 degrees. If the temperature rises above 70.5 degrees, the thermostat automatically activates the air conditioner and cools the air down to 70 degrees. If the temperature goes below 69.5 degrees, the thermostat automatically activates the heater and warms the air to 70 degrees.

Your Mind's *Master Control Center*

Your body has the master blueprint for health located in your DNA. The expression of that master plan is managed by your *Master Control Center* where there is a control for every function of your body, and for every emotion, habit, and skill. Each one of those controls is like a thermostat with a specific value as its set-point. Your body operates automatically in the tight range around the set-point on each control.

Your home thermostat acts like an automatic pilot for your temperature. Your attention is not required once you set the set-point. Similarly, your body function controls are also automatic, with no attention necessary to keep them at their set-point. Adjustments are automatically made without your conscious thought to maintain each of your body's functions. The tight range around the function set-point is automatically maintained by your control as it triggers the appropriate adjustments in the body. Your mind's *Master Control Center* is in charge of every aspect of your body-mind.

Also, just as the thermostat has a method (usually a knob) to make adjustments to the temperature set-point, each control in your *Master Control Center* has an adjustment that lets you move the set-point up or down. Your mind is always monitoring performance against the set-point on each of your controls. When you make a set-point change on one of your controls, your mind-body automatically makes the necessary adjustments to keep that specific function aligned with your new set-point.

Your Subconscious Control Center

The Control Center technique seems to work magically because the miracle is that your subconscious runs your body on autopilot. The second miracle is that your subconscious takes commands from your imagination just as easily as it takes them from your memory and actual

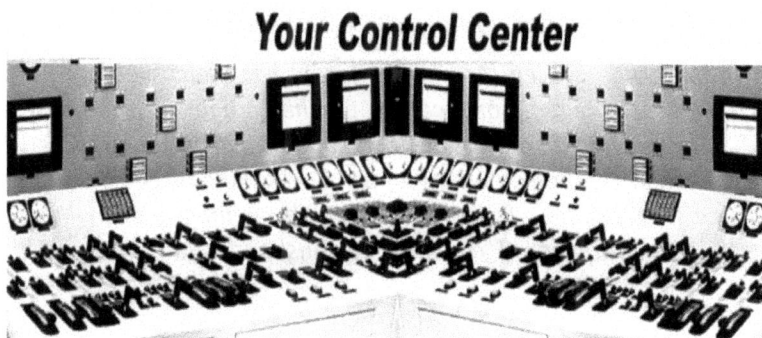

Your Control Center

physical input from your senses. For your subconscious mind, all are equally real! Therefore, an adjustment on your imaginary control is just as real as the objects you are seeing with your eyes and touching with your fingers! An imagined adjustment is just as effective as if you were manipulating a physical adjustment knob in your hand!

Control Center Experiences

You can go into your *Master Control Center* and turn down any discomfort. You can even turn discomfort off completely and forever banish it. I have helped hundreds of people do this. You can accomplish the same thing! Let me repeat that, and just let the importance sink in:

"You can go into your mind's *Master Control Center* and turn down, even turn off, any discomfort you may have!"

Here is what some of my students who used the Control Center technique report:

I had comprehensive laser dermatology on my face and arms that went wrong. Since then I have had excruciating pain in my face and arms. I have tried many things to remedy my pain with little or no effect. As a last resort, I found Duncan Tooley, a pain hypnotist in Los Angeles. The results seem unbelievable after a single one-hour Skype session with Duncan. It's almost like a magic spell. I have no pain. I have my old life back able to do everything I want pain-free. --Rebecca Harris

I had some unidentified skin disorder that sent shooting pain whenever my scalp or face was touched. I had to sleep upright because lying on a pillow was so painful that I could not sleep. I also had red bumps on my upper back. Duncan Tooley taught me how to turn off the pain, calm the itching, and make the bumps disappear. I can kiss my husband again without his beard causing pain. I sleep normally on a pillow again. I had no idea that I could easily have control over my pain. --Dina Wiley

Let me repeat one more time. "You can go into your *Master Control Center* and turn down, even turn off completely, any discomfort you may have!" Let's begin!

Control Center Comfort Adjustment

A unique feature of your mind's *Master Control Center* is that all the controls are arranged as opposite (inverse) pairs. When one control is adjusted downward, its related control is adjusted upward. The effect of each control is the same, only the representation is different. For example, the opposite of **insomnia** is **restful sleep**. In our mind's Master Control Center there is a control pair for these opposites, as shown in the following diagram.

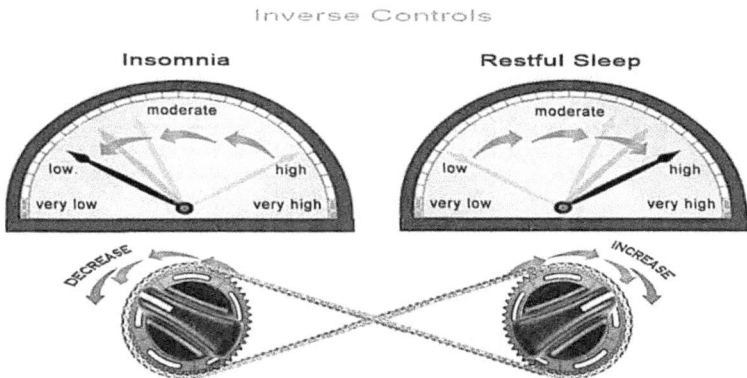

Inverse Controls

Insomnia

Restful Sleep

When you decrease insomnia by rotating the *Insomnia* control knob counterclockwise, the *Insomnia* needle moves to the left and lower. The gearing of the control knobs causes the *Restful Sleep* control knob to rotate clockwise, moving the *Restful Sleep* needle to the right and higher. The needles indicate the new set-points for your types of sleep.

Simulate rotating the knob and the needle movement now on the diagram by pretending that the knobs are real physical objects that you grab and turn. Notice that both dials change whenever one of the knobs is turned. Notice how rotating the *Restful Sleep* control knob clockwise will rotate the *Insomnia* control knob counterclockwise. Turning *Restful Sleep* **UP** simultaneously turns *Insomnia* **DOWN.**

Similarly, you have a *Comfort* control that is paired with a *Discomfort* control in your mind's *Master Control Center.* Because the subconscious works more effectively with positives than negatives, you will focus on turning up the *Comfort* control rather than turning down the *Discomfort (P@#$)* control. Your *Discomfort* control will automatically be turned down because of its inverse connection to your *Comfort* control.

Steps to Use Your Master Control Center for Relief

Step 1. Prepare Your Chart.

Use a *Comfort Control Chart* like the one below to plan your adjustment.

Use a pencil so that you can make changes if needed. You can mark directly in the book, but perhaps a better idea is to download and print a copy of the diagram below, from the book extras website: *www.feelgreat.duncantooley.com*

Select one area of your body that has been getting your attention with some discomfort that you desire to eliminate. Write the name of that area in the blank on the first line of your *Comfort Control Chart.*

My _____ (area of body) **COMFORT CONTROL CHART**

My Intention:_____

Affirmations:

1._____

2._____

3._____

Afformation (Question)

4._____

Say each 10x as you fall asleep and on first awakening.

Step 2. Set Your Intention.

Think about WHY you want to eliminate the discomfort from that area of your body. What is your end result that is motivating your desire for this comfort change? Formulate your intention for making the change in a positive way that includes the reason or expectation about how an improved comfort adjustment will affect your life.

How will your life be different afterward and why do you seek that difference? What will you do that you don't or can't do now? Write your intention on the *Intention* line of your *Comfort Control Chart.*

Once you have written your intention, edit it with a critical eye to be sure that your intention contains only things that you desire. Omit negative words like "no," "never," "none," or "won't." Remove words that denote anything not pleasing to you. Continue to edit and improve your intention until you are satisfied that your written intention expresses the real WHY behind your desire.

Step 3. Plan Your Adjustment.

- On the dials, the needle comes from bottom center up to the outer arc like a speedometer needle. Draw the missing needle on the *DISCOMFORT* dial in the position that shows your most frequent discomfort level in that area of your body. This is your initial discomfort set-point.

- Decide how low you want your future *DISCOMFORT* set-point to be. This could be *low, very low,* or all the way *OFF.*

- Simulate grabbing the control knob and slowly turning the knob counter-clockwise, imagining the needle moving to the left and lower as you turn the knob. Stop turning when the needle reaches your desired new position.

- Mark another needle on the dial showing your desired new set-point where the needle stopped as you were decreasing.

- Draw some curved arrows on the face of the dial starting from your original needle position to your ending needle position.

- Now repeat the process by marking your corresponding *COMFORT* dial to show the corresponding opposite effect. (Hint: if you marked the *DISCOMFORT* control starting needle as "high," the corresponding *COMFORT* control starting needle is pointing to "low.")

104

- Physically try to grasp the *COMFORT* control knob and turn the knob clockwise as you imagine your comfort needle moving right and higher. Mark the position of your new *COMFORT* level needle in its final high position. Mark the curved arrows on the dial face from the original needle position to your new higher set-point needle position.

Step 4. Formulate Your Affirmations.

Affirmations are short messages to your subconscious. They are used to reaffirm what you believe or to reinforce a change you are implanting. They work by the Law of Attraction, the most powerful Natural Law. The Law of Attraction can be stated as:

"What you think about (believe & tell yourself) is what you get (is attracted to you)."

"What you think about, comes about!"

- Formulate three affirmations that reinforce your new comfort level that results from your adjustment. Word them to affirm that the comfort has *already* happened. As you mentally formulate each affirmation, validate your wording against the guidelines for affirmation structure from Step 1 in Chapter 11, Affirmations.
- Write your affirmations on lines 1-3 under the knobs on your Comfort Control Chart.

Step 5. Formulate Your Afformation.

- Formulate a question whose answer is unknown to you and whose answer reinforces your intention and your increased comfort. Your question should engage your mind to start offering possible answers that reinforce the comfort you are increasing! Your mind is already radiating *comfort-focused* energy! (See Chapter 11, *Affirmation-Afformation*, for structuring afformations.)
- Write your afformation on your *Comfort Control Chart* line 4.

Step 6. Review (and possibly edit) Your Chart.

- Take a good look at your new set-point position, your intention, your affirmations, and your afformation question. Ask yourself, "Are these all consistent, work together, and in my best interest?"

- Review your affirmations against the composition criteria and edit as necessary. Does your afformation ask a question about how or why the change has taken place?

- After you have honed these elements to be just right, say your affirmations aloud 5 times. Then ask your afformation question 5 times.

*** *Note: Steps 7, 8, & 9 are performed with your eyes closed.* Therefore, study these three steps, and then perform them from memory.

Step 7. Enter Your Master Control Center.

It is time to actually make your adjustment. You will do this by using the *Visualization* technique. (Review that technique now in Chapter 10 if needed.)

- Reread your intention.

- Memorize your affirmations and afformation.

- Close your eyes.

- Invoke your *Relaxation Response* by deep breathing and muscle relaxation. (See Chapter 4 for refresher if needed.)

- Imagine yourself at your favorite place in Nature, being there 100% in all your senses and enjoying every aspect of that place very much.

- Imagine going into your *Master Control Center.* You may find your Control Center in a cabin or tent at your favorite place. Perhaps a magical being brings your Control Center to you on a flying carpet, or perhaps the genie that emerges from the lamp you found shows you where to find your Master Control Center. However you choose to imagine it, get yourself to your Master Control Center, go inside, and be awestruck by the vast array of controls.

Step 8. Locate Your Comfort Control.

- Find the linked pair of controls for your *DISCOMFORT* and *COMFORT* among the many controls in your Master Control Center. (They may be in the control section for muscles, or for emotions, or some other section depending on your type of discomfort. You will know where it is located once you enter your Master Control Center).

- Position yourself in front of the controls and notice how the needles read exactly as you had drawn them on your Comfort Control Chart.

- Feel the excitement of every cell in your body in anticipation of how much better you will be feeling and how much happier.

Step 9. Make Your Adjustment.

- A. Grasp the COMFORT Control with your dominant hand.

- B. Slowly turn the control clockwise and watch the needles move. The *COMFORT* needle moves right and higher as the *DISCOMFORT* needle moves left and lower. Stop when the *COMFORT* needle is as high as you desire it to go.

- C. Say your affirmations and afformation (as best as you can remember them with your eyes still closed).

- D. Tell every cell in your body to take note of your new set-points. Let the images of new positions on your dials make an indelible imprint on your mind. Tell your cells to do whatever their function is to maintain your new set-points. Thank them for everything they do for you.

- E. Slowly bring your awareness back to your surroundings and open your eyes.

Step 10. Notice the Difference.

Over the next days and weeks, notice the difference in how you feel. Keep a record and write your own miracle story.

> ***Pro-Tip:*** The *Master Control Center* technique that you have just completed has wide applicability because there is a control for every aspect of your life. You can use the control center process to make adjustments to emotions, food preferences, stress, habits, and skills. Controls are useful for turning down habits that you want to discontinue and for increasing habits that you desire to acquire or strengthen. Controls exist for turning up academic skills, business/professional skills, athletic skills, and social/relationship skills.
>
> When you imagine the specific control for whatever you desire to adjust, you will easily find that control in your *Master Control Center* and successfully adjust it by using this technique.

> ***Stories:*** The Control Center is at the heart of my weight loss programs. Clients who used the Control Center technique for eating/drinking issues reported:
>
> *"I used to drink 5 cokes every day. After turning my coke control off last week, I only drank one all week."* --Lou Ann
>
> *"I used to eat a platter of French fries and then get a refill. Now that I turned my French fry control down, they just don't taste that great anymore. If my restaurant food comes with French fries, I eat one or two and that is all."* --Aaron
>
> *"I turned off my wine control because I couldn't stop drinking two or more glasses of wine each evening. That was sabotaging my weight control efforts. After I turned my wine preference control off, I totally stopped drinking wine."*—Kathy

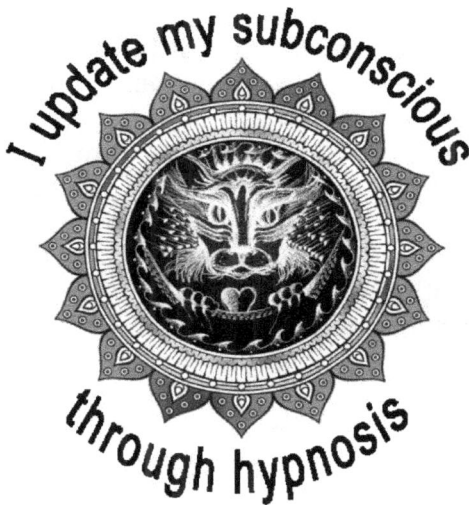

Chapter 13

Hypnosis

About Hypnosis

Hypnosis is a natural state of awareness that you already experience every day. You enter a trance state when you day-dream, meditate, listen to rhythmic instrumental music, just before falling asleep, upon awakening, and when engaged in semi-automatic behavior such as freeway driving or athletic activity labeled as being *in the zone.*

Clinical (Therapeutic) Hypnosis

Hypnosis has long been used to help the body cure illnesses. *Sleep temples* are documented in Egypt, Greece, Rome, England, and India, where healing hypnosis was induced by *priest-doctors.* Clinical (therapeutic) hypnosis is a professionally accepted stand-alone alternative wellness modality that does not require a state license. Clinical hypnosis is self-regulated through professional certification associations. The AMA (American Medical Association) has endorsed numerous studies documenting the medical benefits of hypnosis. Many hospitals now employ hypnotists on their staff to assist patient healing. Hundreds of thousands, perhaps millions, of smokers have quit instantly using hypnosis.

Clinical hypnosis is used for beneficial change. It is totally different than the entertainment hypnosis of TV, movies, and stage shows.

Performance Hypnosis

Performance hypnosis is used by athletes, students, and many successful people to improve and augment their performance. Sporting competitions are won first in the athlete's mind that controls the performance of the body. The same is true with life skills, academic success, focus, creativity, and other skill-stretching situations. Learning self-hypnosis to use on oneself in life's challenging moments is a powerful success factor.

Why Hypnosis Works

Hypnosis works because of the way your mind works. Put very simply, your subconscious mind, that part below the surface and relatively inaccessible, runs your body, emotions, and habits, mostly on a type of autopilot program. That's a lot of your life! When you want to change something about your body, emotions, or habits, your conscious mind wants to stay in control and blocks your access to your subconscious. Hypnosis permits distraction of your conscious mind so that you can give your subconscious effective suggestions that are readily accepted. Once accepted, the subconscious automatically applies the suggestions and produces the desired adjustment in your body, emotions, or habits.

Hypnosis produces a pleasant and relaxed inner feeling that provides a direct path to the deeper regions of your mind and consciousness. Hypnosis permits you to remember things previously forgotten, to moderate your emotions, to mitigate any physical dis-ease, to overcome your limitations, to turn off discomfort, and to transform yourself into an unlimited human! The transformation power of hypnosis comes from accessing the power that results from the junction of your mind, your body, and your spirit (with its access to Infinite Wisdom).

Visualization, mental rehearsal, contemplative prayer, yoga, Reiki massage, chanted prayers, ceremonial dancing, repetitive drumbeats, and music, all contain elements of hypnosis, which is sometimes called guided meditation.

> *Story:* My friend, Rhona, works with doctors at five clinics where she assists clients with their physical and medical issues by using both *guided imagery* and *hypnosis*. Imagery is the language of the body ("Feel the blood flow") and hypnosis is the language of the mind ("Know that you have control over every cell and wellness is occurring").

Hypnosis for Pain

Hypnosis was the standard method for reducing pain during surgery before chloroform and ether came into wide use for anesthesia. Hypnosis was the normal anesthesia for surgery on soldiers during the Civil War. Today, thousands of surgeries and births are performed painlessly without drugs by use of hypnosis as anesthesia.

> *"Hypnosis takes the edge off and makes patients feel better. With some, it's dramatic. It works so well they don't need pain medicine at all ... Hypnosis is an astonishingly powerful pain reliever... that seems to be useful for virtually every clinical pain problem imaginable."*-- Dr. David Patterson, MD, University of Washington, Harbor View Burn Center

> *"Pain control techniques using hypnosis are simple, effective, easy to learn, and applicable to most cancer patients in pain."*
> –Dr. Bernie Siegel, MD, Stanford Cancer Center

My Story: I had my umbilical hernia repair surgery in 2008 using self-hypnosis as my general anesthesia. My surgeon was amazed and said he could not tell the difference between me and someone who had the normal general anesthesia. (My complete story is in the Preface).

Many hospitals now use clinical hypnosis to assist patients in their discomfort management and healing.

Study: In a randomized study of 200 women undergoing surgery for breast cancer, those who received a brief hypnosis session before entering the operating room required less anesthesia and pain medication during surgery, and reported less pain, nausea, fatigue, and discomfort after surgery than women who did not receive hypnosis. (Cf. References, Study 4)

Story: My friend, Jackie, had knee replacement surgery on both knees, done at different times. She said, "I was given a guided meditation CD to listen to before the second surgery. That surgery went much better and my recovery was much faster than the first knee surgery."

Hypnosis works no matter what you call it! The CD of guided meditation instructed Jackie's subconscious that her surgery would go well and recovery would be rapid. Every cell in her body got that message and cooperated accordingly!

> ***My Story:*** A branch of hypnosis called *hypno-birthing* or *Hypno-Babies* permits women to birth children with no drugs, no discomfort, and no sweat! I watched my daughter, Dina, give birth at home using self-hypnosis. She was so relaxed and comfortable, and the birth so effortless and natural, that the midwife sitting nearby almost missed it!

Steps to Use Hypnosis for Physical or Emotional Relief

Step 1. Consult a Clinical Hypnotist.

A hypnotist can help you connect with the source of your discomfort and communicate with the source to find relief for physical ailments.

> ***Story:*** "The first time Duncan saw me, I was lying on the office floor because my back hurt so much I couldn't sit or stand. My wife drove me to the appointment because I couldn't. My pain levels were 9 out of 10. Before our session, I believed in the benefits of hypnosis for OTHERS, but I was afraid that it wouldn't work for me."
>
> "Thankfully, I was wrong! At the end of our appointment, I was able to stand and walk out of the room unassisted! My pain level had gone down to a 4! I was astounded!" –Morgan Kramer

The Center for Disease Control says that 85% of illnesses are caused by *emotional issues.* Emotional stress flips your epigenetic switches that control the expression or repression of your DNA. Discomfort resulting from emotion-triggered illness is probably beyond self-help resolution and requires the assistance of a hypnotist to help you find and resolve the emotional basis for your experience of discomfort.

> *Story:* Hypnosis assisted Brian to find the source of his hurt when no doctor could find any because his discomfort was emotion-based. See the dialog of his hypnosis session in the Appendices as *A1. Emotional P@#$ Case Study.*

If you unable to find a local clinical hypnotherapist to assist you with eliminating physical or emotion-based discomfort, send me an email so that I can assist you remotely: *feelgreat@duncantooley.com.* Remote phone and video sessions have proven successful.

Step 2. Learn Self-Hypnosis.

Self-hypnosis is the technique of hypnosis you use to help yourself whenever you need. Self-hypnosis is easy to learn. You easily achieve mastery with only a few repetitions, as recounted by my self-hypnosis class student:

> *Story:* "For ten years, I lived with chronic pain from non-diabetic neuropathy, during which I spent thousands of dollars on every type of alternative therapy including massage, acupuncture, and chiropractic, with no relief. Once I began using the short routine that Duncan teaches, my pain decreased dramatically and I stopped taking 6 Norco (codeine) tablets daily. I am feeling wonderful about getting my life back! My husband and my doctor are both amazed! I tell everyone I meet to go take the class and learn how to help yourself." –Jane Smolens

You can learn self-hypnosis from either live classes or audio-visual materials. For self-hypnosis resources, see **store.duncantooley.com.**

Step 3. Use Recorded Hypnosis Sessions.

Recorded audio sessions provide you the benefits of hypnosis without the physical presence of a hypnotist.

General hypnosis recordings are nearly as effective as those targeted to specific issues. Clients with a variety of different discomfort issues report that my *Feel Great* recorded relief hypnosis session is effective for them. See the resources page at the front or back of the book, or go to ***store.duncantooley.com*** for information.

Still have some questions about hypnosis? See the truth and falsities about hypnosis in *Appendix A7, Hypnosis Myths Busted,* or call me for an honest discussion at 310-832-0830.

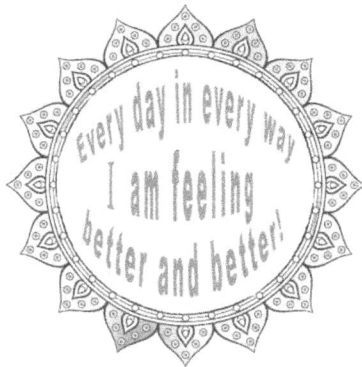

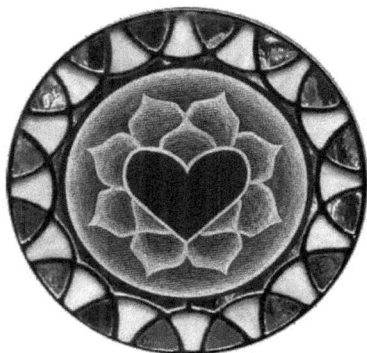

SPIRIT-BASED METHODS TO FEEL GREAT AGAIN

▸ 14. Mantra - Prayer

▸ 15. Mindfulness - Meditation

▸ 16. Yoga

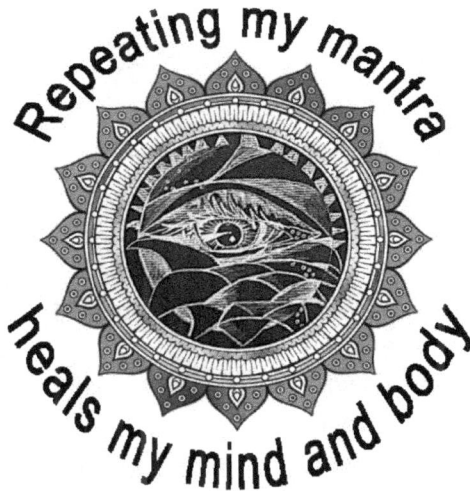

Chapter 14

Mantra - Prayer

About Mantra

A mantra is a word, or group of words, repeated aloud or internally. If the mantra is intended to be heard by a deity, it becomes a prayer. Most religions have some form of prayer bead loop on which you can keep track of the number of repetitions of mantras or prayers.

The words can be repeated as a type of rote chant even without the direct attention of the conscious mind through meditation or mindfulness. Setting an initial intention for the repetition empowers the effectiveness of the rote repetition without further intentionality. The words are effective even in the absence of immediate attention.

Mantras are instructions to your subconscious. The more they are repeated, the greater and quicker the effect they can have.

Steps to Use a Mantra for Relief

Step 1. Select an Appropriate Positive Mantra.

Use an existing word or phrase, or create your own for a specific purpose. Ensure that the words are positive and healing. (See the guidelines in Chapter 11, *Affirmations*). Some mantras are:

- *"Relaxed & Calm."* [implied command to body & mind]
- *"All is well!"* [Implied instruction to body]
- *"Every little cell in my body is happy and well."* [Direct instruction to cells; implies any cells not healthy and well are eliminated and replaced]
- *"Yes! Yes! Yes! Yes! Yes!"* [implied response to all the good the Universe flows to me]
- *"Om Mani Padme Hum."* [Chant of Buddha of Compassion, known by the Chinese as Goddess Kuan Yin. The mantra calms fears, soothes concerns and heals broken hearts.]
- *"Lokah Samastah Sukhino Bhavantu."* [From Jivamukti Yoga School, translates to "May all beings everywhere be happy and free, and may the thoughts, words, and actions of my own life contribute in some way to that happiness and to that freedom for all."]

Step 2. Repeat the Mantra Hundreds of Times.

The mantra is effective for relief because the drone-like repetition puts you into a state of trance, permitting the message of the words to sink deep into that part of your consciousness that controls your body. The more repetitions, the more effective is the process.

~ロ~ロ~ロ~

About Prayer

Prayer brings comfort and uplifting distraction. It builds and maintains an intimate relation with a "greater-than-you-being."

> *Study:* More than half of the 1,204 respondents to a nationwide poll conducted by ABC News, USA Today, and the Stanford University Medical Center said they use prayer against pain. Of those that used prayer, 50% said prayer "worked very well" and another 40% said prayer worked "well." (Cf. Resources, Study 5)

Numerous other studies conclude that people are comforted by religious and spiritual beliefs, activities, and prayer.

If you believe that prayer will help, it definitely will! And the stronger your belief, the more effective prayer will be for relief. Prayer often brings inspiration (sudden thoughts that seem to come from outside of yourself) and terrific results (the stuff of miracles!) that can bring relief and healing.

Steps to Use Prayer for Relief

Step 1. Decide to Whom to Address Your Prayer.

Many names have been given to the greater-than-you-being: God, Allah, Yahweh, Abba, Source Energy, Jehovah, Elohim, I am, Infinite Intelligence, Creator, Divine Being, Lord, Messiah, Savior, Jesus, Krishna, Wakan Tanka, Guanyin, Saraswati ...

If you are a believer in a "greater-than-you-being," use whatever name or phrase you choose, knowing that you are heard. You will join billions of people who find relief through prayer, mantras, and meditation.

Step 2. Choose and Use Your Choice of Prayer Form.

- Create your own spontaneous prayer each time you are moved to pray. An intimate conversation uses spontaneous words, or even no words at all. Mix in the various types of prayer so that your prayer is not just supplication.

- Script a prayer that you subsequently use each time you pray.

- Use words that have been prepared by others to express the universal desire for relief. Here are some:

Prayer for Those in Physical P@#$ by Maureen Pratt

"Help me to feel your calming hand upon me
when I am in P@#$.
Let your ever-loving comfort enfold me,
And give me the heart to see
that in my suffering, I am becoming
closer to you...
and more divine."

Prayer for P@#$ Relief by Jonathan Fashbaugh

"God of the Universe, we worship you and call all of our bodies and minds into alignment with your Kingdom. Your Kingdom is free of P@#$. The P@#$ in our bodies and the emotional P@#$ that some of us are experiencing is not of God. We take authority over this P@#$ and command it to leave."

Psalm 18:2

"The LORD is my rock and my fortress and my deliverer, my God, my rock, in whom I take refuge, my shield, and the strength of my salvation, my stronghold."

Psalm 34:18

"Jehovah is near to the brokenhearted and saves the crushed in spirit."

Hindu Prayer for Wellness
"Om Abed Deya Ahmed"

Buddhist Prayer for Wellness
"I evoke the presence of Great Compassion.
Fill my heart with compassion
for myself and all living things.
We are nourished by the same Source."

Step 3. Communicate.

Keep the conversation going. Use the various types of prayer. Communication is bidirectional; listen as well as speak. The Balinese say "Make a prayer of everything you do."

My Story: When discussing prayer with a friend, she told me something about prayer that I have never forgotten: "I no longer use a prayer of petition. I don't ask for anything. My only prayer is gratitude. God already knows what I need and is already providing it. Asking for it seems doubting and insulting. I simply give thanks for receiving what I need because I know it is already being delivered!"

Pro-Tip: Use these different types of prayer for variety in your conversation:

The prayer of request (or petition, supplication) is the expression of asking for something you want. Will you ask for relief, acceptance, or learning how to control your discomfort?

The prayer of faith is an expression of belief in the greater-than-being and the inherent goodness of that being.

The prayer of worship acknowledges who the greater-than-being is.

The prayer of intercession is a request for others as we intercede for them. Praying for relief of your family member or friend suffering from discomfort is a prayer of this type.

The prayer of thanksgiving (or gratitude) is the natural follow-up of the prayer of supplication, or just thankfulness for blessings received even when not requested. The Psalms are filled with prayers of thanksgiving.

The prayer of consecration is a setting apart for a particular or unique purpose relating to the greater-than-being.

The prayer of appreciation is gratitude for all of nature, for existence and life, for being human with the capacity to enjoy.

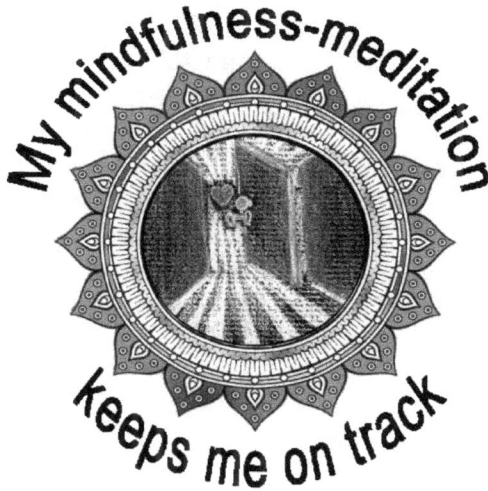

Chapter 15

My mindfulness-meditation keeps me on track

Mindfulness - Meditation

About Mindfulness

Mindfulness is the mental state of purposefully focusing your awareness on the present moment, while calmly acknowledging and non-judgmentally accepting your thoughts, feelings, and bodily sensations as they flow by. Mindfulness is purposely and consciously paying attention. You can implement mindfulness by simply taking a moment to focus attention on your breath. Mindfulness relieves discomfort because it toggles epigenetic switches that control the operation of body functions.

~▫~▫~▫~

About Meditation

Meditation is setting aside time to do something that is beneficial for yourself. Meditation has been shown to stimulate the immune system and even to re-wire the neuron connections in the brain. The brain structure of life-long meditators, for example Tibetan monks, is noticeably different than that of non-meditators. The medical community has long realized that a stressed mind is the enemy of healing and hence recommends any practice that calms the mind and creates positive emotions.

Mindful meditation is a practice of setting aside time to calm the mind and focus only on the present. It sets the stage for a day spent in mindfulness. Even as little as a single day of mindfulness can produce brain function changes.

Mindfulness vs. Mindlessness

You are in the opposite state, mindlessness, when you realize you just ate a candy bar without noticing a single bite, or arrived at your destination without remembering the drive. If you have some discomfort, examine your day for opportunities to be more mindful. Mindfulness will make you feel better! Being mindful lets you:

- Juggle work, home, finances, family, and other conflicting demands
- Hear what your body is trying to tell you
- Stop toxic self-talk, worry, and stress

Study: One study reports that mindfulness meditation can alter behavioral, neural, and biochemical processes.

After 8 hours of mindfulness practice, a group of meditators, compared to a control group, showed a range of genetic and molecular differences, including altered levels of gene-regulating machinery and reduced levels of pro-inflammatory genes, resulting in faster physical recovery from a stressful situation. (Cf. References, Study 6)

Steps to Use Mindful Meditation for Relief

Step 1. Begin with Noticing.

Simply notice what is happening in real time. Mindfulness helps you accept your thoughts and feelings without judging them. When you practice mindfulness, your thoughts tune into what is happening in the present moment without rehashing the past or imagining the future.

Step 2. Add Breathing and Imagery.

Use one of the breathing exercises from *Chapter 4, Relaxation Response*. Then use the imagery exercise to relax further.

Step 3. Add Guided Meditation.

From your skills gained in *Chapter 10, Visualization*, expand the scene into observing everything from a totally nonjudgmental attitude. Guided Meditation is so important to a successful mindfulness practice that the Dalai Lama considers guided meditation as the "training wheels" for mindfulness.

Step 4. Make Daily Mindful Meditation a Habit.

Mindfulness can be a vital component of your comfort solution. Mindful meditation is a habit and skill developed over time and with practice. Just a few minutes daily of mindful meditation is mind training at its best. The mental skill that you develop with a daily practice of mindfulness alone, or with meditation, enhances your other comfort-generating techniques and combats nuisance discomfort.

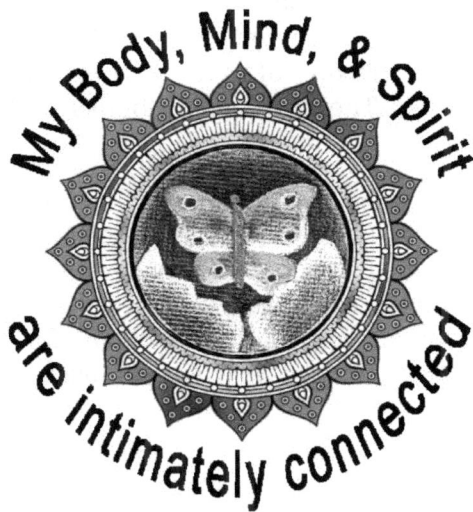

Chapter 16

My Body, Mind, & Spirit are intimately connected

Yoga

About Yoga

It's no secret that yoga increases muscular flexibility and strength, but perhaps you did not know that yoga is a proven treatment for back discomfort, knee discomfort, carpal tunnel syndrome, and other chronic discomfort conditions. Yoga also helps you feel more comfortable in both your mind and your body, thereby easing the stress, anxiety, and depression that can create and reinforce discomfort.

This is logical because yoga invokes the Relaxation Response, a key component of regaining control of your body and mind. Yoga emphasizes breathing and clearing the mind, two other techniques that have already been mentioned. Yoga goes beyond these techniques by adding the tensing and relaxing of muscles through the easy-to-remember poses. There are many books and articles on yoga for discomfort relief.

> **Study:** In a survey of 2,700 people who therapeutically used yoga 2 hours a week for at least a year, reported improvement was 98% for back-pain sufferers, 90% for arthritis/rheumatic disorder sufferers, 80% for those with migraines, and 96% for those with neuromuscular and neurological diseases (Cf. References, Study 7)

> **Study:** In a randomized controlled clinical trial of yoga for neck pain vs. self-care with exercise for neck pain, the pain at rest was reduced by 71% for those who took 10 weeks of yoga. A reduction of 18% was achieved by those in the self-care/exercise group. Yoga led to superior pain relief and functional improvements. The study concluded that yoga appears to be an effective treatment for chronic neck pain with possible additional effects on psychological well-being and quality of life. (Cf. References, Study 8)

Steps to Use Yoga for Relief

Step 1. Take Some Yoga Classes

Taking a yoga class is probably the best way to start. Not only will you become familiar with the proper form for the yoga stretching and balance poses, you are also encouraged by doing it along with others. Since there are many styles of yoga, learn about the ones in your area and choose the most compatible for your introduction to yoga.

Step 2. Do Your Poses at Home Daily.

For many people, yoga each day converts discomfort to comfort and helps them feel great! Yoga may be the perfect thing for you. Even if you do a regular yoga program once or twice a week, doing some poses each day, especially in the morning, will help you feel even better. Using a DVD of a yoga session is an easy way to stay focused and complete your routine.

Step 3. Include Yoga in Your Comfort Solution.

The balance of mind, body, and spirit inherit in a yoga practice makes yoga a great component for your life-long comfort solution. Determine the way you will integrate the beneficial effects of yoga into your life for the long term.

> *Pro-Tip:* Yoga offered for those recovering from cancer, illness, or injuries is usually simpler and more forgiving. It may be suitable no matter your age or beginning physical condition when you first begin yoga.

> *My Story:* In all my life, I had never tried yoga. Because my wife, Dona, transitioned from cancer, I was eligible to take the free yoga classes at the local cancer support center. I began with one class per week and then increased to several days each week as I enjoyed the resulting increase in strength, balance, and flexibility.

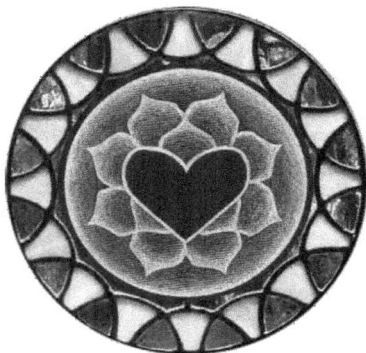

FUN-BASED METHODS TO FEEL GREAT AGAIN

▶ **17. Laughter**

▶ **18. Enjoy -**
    Sing-Play-Write-Paint-Dance

▶ **19. Feel Great Word Search**

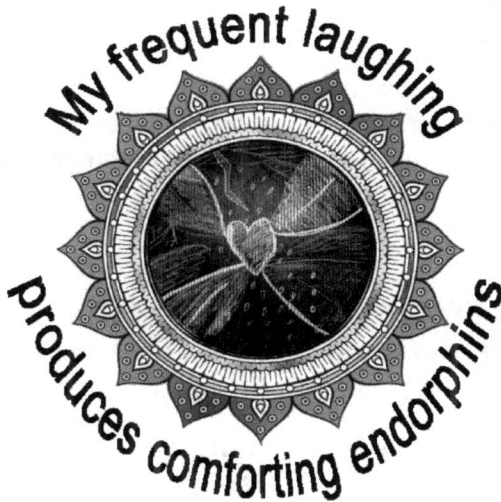

Chapter 17

My frequent laughing produces comforting endorphins

Laughter

About Laughter

Laughter is the quickest, least expensive, always-available discomfort reliever. Your brain is a pharmaceutical chemical factory that produces endorphins when you laugh. Endorphins are a class of chemicals whose name is derived from "endogenous morphine," which means morphine produced by the body.

Make laughing work for you right now by searching your memory for the funniest thing that you ever heard or saw or did. When you retrieve it, have a good laugh! Then refile that memory in your brain's database under the category "instant discomfort reliever." That way you will be able to retrieve that memory instantly when you next want to feel better.

Many studies have been produced on the curative and pain-relieving effects of laughter. Try laughter for yourself. I'll wager that you can't have a good laugh and still feel like a victim of discomfort.

Steps to Use Laughter for Relief

Step 1. Use Your Memory.
Recall the funniest thing that you every heard or saw or did. Have a good laugh over it, and then repeat.

Step 2. Use the Laugh Formula.
A way to get a good laugh going is to use the formula that laughing is just the "H" sound on the front of each of the vowels:

> *"Ha, ha, ha, ha, ha, ha, ha!"*
> *"He, he, he, he, he, he, he!"*
> *"Hi, hi, hi, hi, hi, hi, hi!"*
> *"Ho, ho, ho, ho, ho, ho, ho!"*
> *"Hu, hu, hu, hu, hu, hu, hu!"*
> *"Isn't that funny?"*

Step 3. Use the Internet.
Find and watch videos of funny things that make you laugh, like compilations of dogs or cats doing astounding tricks. Search for and watch the 50 funniest YouTube videos.

> ***My Story:*** I used self-hypnosis as my general anesthesia in 2008 for an umbilical hernia repair. Everything had been progressing fine until the surgeon began to pull the stitches tight and my discomfort level increased. I

knew I had to do something to stay motionless, so I began to laugh to produce endorphins to lower my discomfort. The laughing worked! Meanwhile, I wondered if the surgeon and his assistant were thinking I was crazy for laughing as they pulled the stitches tighter. I discovered later that my face was under a blue tent and no one could see me laughing. (Read the entire story in the Preface).

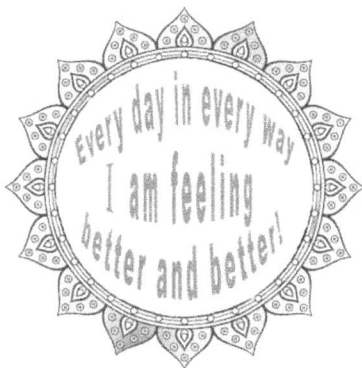

Every day in every way
I am feeling
better and better!

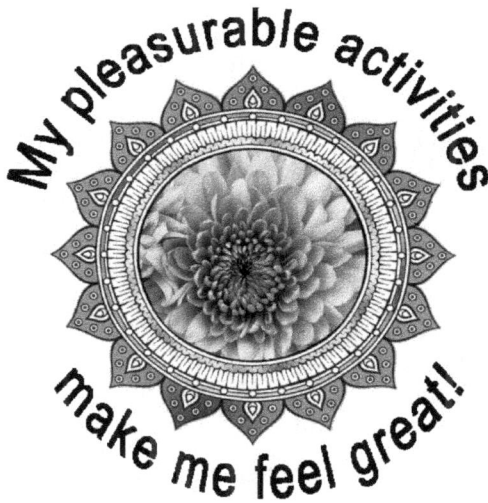

Chapter 18

Enjoy-Sing-Play-Write-Paint-Dance

About Enjoy

Enjoying anything that you regard as beautiful provides relief from discomfort for two reasons:

- Your brain releases dopamine, the brain's pleasure chemical that makes you feel good.

- You are distracted from the discomfort because your brain can only focus on one thing at a time.

You have probably experienced that a walk outdoors in a park or in a nature setting feels good and energizes your mind, body, and spirit. Likewise, enjoying pleasurable art, listening to soothing music, being absorbed in a great novel, or having a fun hobby are all useful in reducing discomfort.

Recognition of the healing effects of enjoying beauty has led to art programs in 45 percent of the country's health care institutions (2009 report by the Global Alliance for Arts and Health). These are predominantly through art displays and performances, bedside activities, art carts, and healing gardens. For example, the Cleveland Clinic's 27 locations house some 5,000 pieces of art.

> ***Study:*** Research coordinated by the neurological and psychiatric sciences department at the University of Bari, Italy, found that looking at beautiful art lowers pain levels in hospital patients. (Cf. References, Study 9)

> ***Study:*** Brain scans conducted at McGill University reveal that listening to pleasing music increases activity in parts of the brain's reward center, releasing the brain chemical dopamine. The more pleasing the listeners found the music to be, the less pain they felt. (Cf. References, study 10)

Steps to Use Enjoyment for Relief

Step 1. Select Your Enjoyable Music.

Decide on the favorite music that you enjoy. Keep the CD or mp3 of it available. Listen to it whenever you want to feel better. Have it on your phone so you can listen anytime with some earbuds.

Step 2. Select Your Favorite Nature Setting Nearby.

Have a place that you can go when you need a dose of Nature's medicine of beauty. It could be a park, a rural setting, your backyard. Find a place where you can witness the sunset, check the local sunset time, get outside a few minutes before, and wait for the pink magic afterwards.

Step 3. Select Your Home Artworks.

Have in your home one or more works of art that are peaceful and soothing. Some homes have a painted or wallpaper mural of a nature scene that provide subconscious comfort just by seeing them. Consider covering a wall with a scene you really like.

Decorate your home with prints, posters, or original works of art that move you. Select them as objects that will relax you and cause the pleasure response just by focusing on their beauty. Then they will always be available for you when you desire relief.

> **Extra:** The book extras website has a colored mandala mosaic of a sunrise that can brighten any décor. You may freely use it to brighten your day as wallpaper on your computer or phone, or as a wall or refrigerator decoration. Get it at: *www.feelgreat.duncantooley.com*

Step 4. Turn Your Hobby into a Passion.

If you have a hobby the gives you enjoyment, indulge yourself in it more fully. Turn to it whenever you need more comfort. You will be amazed at how good it feels!

Scrapbooking, doodling, collecting, reading, movies, fishing, gardening, walking, shopping, sewing, golf, bicycling, pet care, crafting, playing cards, hiking, cooking, restaurant sampling, writing, bowling, painting, running, dancing, theater, billiards, lazing at the beach, or volunteering. Whatever your hobby, do more of it for relief.

Step 5. Meet with Your Friends.

Pleasure comes from being in social situations that are enjoyable and distracting. Form a group that meets regularly for tea and comradery, lunch, or an outing. (Caution: Choose only individuals who keep the conversation positive and only on pleasant topics.)

~◻~◻~◻~

About Singing

Singing and the melodious sound that singing makes has a therapeutic effect and will decrease discomfort. There is an entire profession of musical therapy that assists persons to heal through creative sound-making with musical instruments or their voice. Actively creating sound with your voice has a stronger effect than just receptively enjoying music; it stimulates your emotions, especially joy, which releases endorphins.

> ***Study:*** A 2004 study of chronic pain patients showed they experienced pain relief not just when singing, but for a long time afterward. Patients in the study were divided into two groups: some attended nine 30-minute group singing sessions. Others were sent to exercise sessions accompanied by music for the same number of sessions and length of time. Patients in the singing group reported significant pain reduction, not just immediately after the sessions, but at 6 months afterward. (Cf. References, Study 11)

Steps to Use Singing for Relief

Step 1. Use Your Voice.

Singing sends energy out of your body. Singing causes your brain to focus on the song, thereby producing a distraction from discomfort. Knowing the words to a song is not essential. You can sing a melody without words. You can make up your own tune or your own words. You can hum along with the radio or a recording.

Step 2. Enter Your Song Experience in Your Journal.

Make a notation of what you sang or hummed and how you felt. It will serve as a reminder to do it more often. Experiment with lyrics without a tune; pretend it is poetry.

~ ❏ ~ ❏ ~ ❏ ~

About Play

The definition of play is "engage in activity for enjoyment and recreation rather than a serious or practical purpose."

Play can be anything that fits that definition, from playing cards, to playing video games, to playing a musical instrument, to playing sports, even just being together and playing with a friend.

Steps to Use Play for Relief

Step 1. Play Making Sound

If you have a musical instrument that you play, now is the time to use it to make some noise. Even if you haven't played it recently, the brain activity from playing the instrument will be comforting.

If you don't play a musical instrument, don't try to learn an instrument for relief; instead feel free to make your own creative sound on any noisemaker without any rules, comparison, or judgement.

Anything that makes sound can be used as a musical instrument for relief. With two pencils, every solid object becomes a drum. Several spoons together make a metallic percussion sound that you can beat out easily on soft or hard surfaces. Set your imagination loose on creating other instruments and sounds, and notice how much better you feel!

Step 2. Play a Video Game.

Medical studies have shown the immersive video games, especially virtual reality games reduce the perception of discomfort in a manner that can be observed in live brain scans (fMRI). Give it a try! It is interesting that a study found that seniors who played video games reported being happier than those who did not, although no causal connection has been determined. (Cf. References, Study 35)

Step 3. Play Any Game.

Play any kind of game. Play a game with yourself like a crossword puzzle, a logic problem, or an on-line game. Play a game with someone else; a card game, or board game, or a sport like table tennis. If you are more athletically inclined, make it a game of tennis, or basketball, or just basketball "HORSE."

~◻~◻~◻~

About Write

Scientific evidence supports that writing (or journaling) provides health and psychological benefits. The act of writing accesses your left brain, which is analytical and rational. While your left brain is occupied, your right brain is free to create, intuit and feel.

Keeping a journal allows you to track patterns, trends, improvement, and growth over time.

Your journaling will be most effective if you do it daily for 15-20 minutes. Begin anywhere, and forget spelling and punctuation. Write quickly, as this frees your brain from rules, inhibitions, and other blocks. Beyond that, there are no rules about what you write. Your journal is an all-accepting, nonjudgmental friend where you can tell all and express your inmost feelings, hopes, plans, and frustrations. The process results in a great sense of comfort and satisfaction.

Steps to Use Writing for Relief

Step 1. Acquire a Journal.

This can be a simple notebook or something fancy, whatever pleases you. A simple school composition book works fine. For added enjoyment, dress it up with a decorated cover or by pasting a photo on it.

Step 2. Write Daily.

Set a time, place, and duration. Then follow your those every day. Let whatever is on your mind that day flow out of your body through your arm, hand, pen or pencil. Let it also be a record of your comfort level.

Step 3. Look Back.

After you have been journaling for a while, it's fun to look back at what you wrote a month, a year, or a few years previously. It's pleasing to see how far you have come.

~□~□~□~

About Paint

Paint is the term I use here to represent art-making of any type. It could be painting, drawing, molding clay, wood carving, or even sewing, knitting, quilt-making or cake decorating.

Making art is a proven method for generating pleasure-producing neurotransmitters as well as providing mental distraction. Studies have shown that painting and drawing can relieve pain and lower stress. That is why many hospitals have creative art activities for their patients. It is also one reason why adult coloring books are now popular.

Steps to Use Painting for Relief

Step 1. Acquire Your Art Materials.

Start with something easy. Get an adult coloring book and some crayons, colored pencils, or pens. Each page typically gives satisfaction after a few minutes of coloring. A paint-by-number picture is good if you are planning on plenty of time. Perhaps you desire an unstructured creativity where you create your own designs. For this, drawing pads or sketch books are a great choice along with colored pencils, pens, pastels, or crayons.

Extra: The mandala images from this book have been pulled together into a free coloring book that you can use for your art activity. Get the *Mandala Coloring Book* at: *www.feelgreat.duncantooley.com.*

Step 2. Make Your Art!

You are making art whenever you create something. It doesn't matter how others might evaluate your creation. You are making it for yourself and for your own comfort. Be bold! Make your own rules about what it should be.

Pro-Tip: An art form that is easy, fun, and totally mind-engaging is what I call "P-Kazo Doodle" paintings. They start with a doodle-scribble of a few lines. Then the creative challenge is to turn them into something recognizable with the fewest additional lines. The painting is finished by coloring the areas enclosed by the lines. The result looks like a stained glass window with the image resembling the works of Pablo Picasso with exaggerated but recognizable features. That's why I call them *P-Kazo* paintings. To see some of mine, go to www.tooleyartstudio.com/p-kazo-paintings

~ ❑ ~ ❑ ~ ❑ ~

About Dance

Dance is to move rhythmically in a pattern. Any type of dance can be therapeutic and comforting. Dance therapy improves self-esteem, attentiveness, body image, and communication skills. Dance reduces stress, fears, anxieties, isolation, chronic discomfort, and depression. Dance enhances the body's circulatory and respiratory system functions.

Tai chi is a very slow structured form of dance that helps ease discomfort. Regular, ongoing tai chi sessions confer the most benefit.

Study: Sixty-six people with fibromyalgia were divided randomly into two groups: one group took tai chi classes twice a week, the other group attended wellness education and stretching sessions twice a week. After 12 weeks, those in the tai chi group reported less pain, fewer depression symptoms, and better sleep than the control group. (Cf. References, Study 12)

Steps to Use Dancing for Relief

Step 1. Dancing at Home.

Put on your favorite dance music and dance around the house. Feel the exhilaration! Be free! Forget everything else! Notice how good your feel! Put dancing in your to-do list or calendar for each day to get it off to a great start.

Step 2. Go Out Dancing.

Go somewhere to dance where others are also dancing. It could be line dancing, a club, or a friend's party. Just dance! An alternative is to go to a friend's house and just the two of you dance there.

Step 3. Take a Dance Class.

Take a line dancing, Hawaiian hula dancing, or a belly-dancing class. Have fun with others as you learn dance moves you can do by yourself at home whenever you choose.

Think of tai chi as a really slow dance. Join a class that meets weekly. After the class is over, continue to do your tai chi exercises at home or with others weekly.

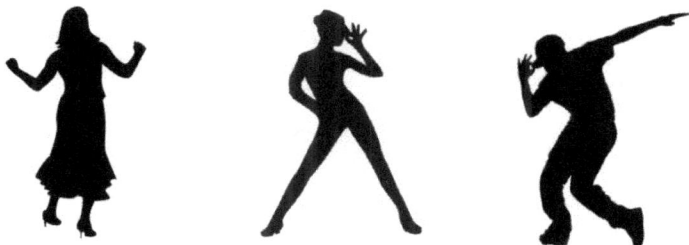

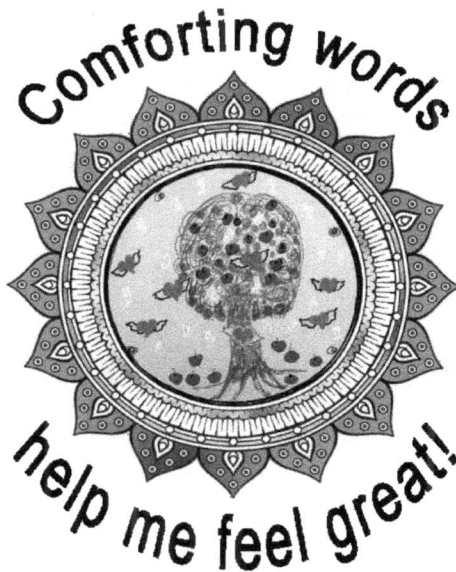

Chapter 19

Feel Great Word Search

About Feel Great Word Search

The *Feel Great Word Search* technique is a recent protocol based on how the subconscious mind works, the importance of language, and the use of positive affirmations. Scientific evidence of the performance of the word-search method for feeling great is not yet available. Just use the fun technique and discover how well it works for you!

Feel Great Word Search Puzzle

(See instructions on opposite page →)

SWITCH IT OFF

BETTER EACH DAY

COMFORTABLE I AM

COMFORT THOUGHTS

HOPE ABOUNDS

I DESERVE COMFORT

FREEDOM NOW

JOYFUL MIND

MIND HEALS BODY

MINE IS HEALTH

RELAXED RELIEF

MIND RUNS MY BODY

FEEL GREAT

CELEBRATE LIFE

FEEL GREAT RELIEF

FEELING GREATEST

FEELING OF JOY

FEEL WONDERFUL

GREAT FEELING NOW

LAUGH EVERY DAY

A BETTER BODY STORY

POSITIVE MIND

STRONG MIND POWER

```
F E E L I N G O F J O Y N Z D I B I
F Y U Q J R E L A X E D R E L I E F
S D N U O B A E P O H J A Q P T T L
L C Y M M A W O N M O D E E R F T A
S T H G U O H T T R O F M O C E E U
F T U W O N G N I L E E F T A E R G
Z V T O N J O Y F U L M I N D L E H
M I N D H E A L S B O D Y Y O I A E
Z D U F F O T I H C T I W S B N C V
F E I L E R T A E R G L E E F G H E
O P O S I T I V E M I N D F D G D R
M C O M F O R T A B L E I A M R A Y
Z E F I L E T A R B E L E C Z E Y D
Y R O T S Y D O B R E T T E B A C A
D T R E W O P D N I M G N O R T S Y
W Y D O B Y M S N U R D N I M E C F
L I F E E L W O N D E R F U L S E F
E E T P Z M I N E I S H E A L T H B
```

Steps to Use Feel Great Word Search Puzzle for Relief

Phrases have spaces removed and can be positioned in any of 8 directions in the letter-block. The steps for puzzle solution are designed to maximize the comfort-producing effect:

1. Read this entire set of instructions before you start.
2. Be in a relaxed, plenty-of-time setting.
3. Read the word list out loud slowly.
4. Read the word list again aloud from the bottom up.
5. Close your eyes and see how many words or phrases you can remember.
6. Repeat reading the word list aloud in both directions until you can say at least 10 from memory.
7. Scan each row of letters from left to right, and then back from right to left. Your subconscious will be solving the puzzle and applying the positive concepts of the words to your body and your life.
8. Circle the matching words and phrases that appear. Cross the found items off the word list.
9. Scan down a column and then back up, one column at a time.
10. Read the word list again, focusing on the ones still missing. All words are present!
11. With a straight-edge, examine each diagonal line of letters in both directions and both 45° angles.
12. Memorize the words still missing and put the puzzle aside for some time, like a few hours, or a day.
13. Say your memorized missing words out loud at least 5 times during your break interval. Tune your mind to find the words next time.

14. When you resume, gaze at the entire block of letters, asking your mind to find the missing words.

15. If words are still unfound after 2 minutes, continue with the next step to enter the last phase of the search.

16. Select a pair of adjacent letters from the word(s), for example, if the phrase *Feelings of Joy* was still not found, you could select the adjacent pair of letters *J* and *O*.

17. Scan the entire letter block to find every *J*. Examine each of the 8 letters around each *J* looking for an *O*. When found, examine the other letters in the same direction as the *O* for a *Y* and then the entire word or phrase. You will certainly find them all with this last process.

Note: Only use the adjacent-letter-pair method as your last resort. The adjacent letter process bypasses the power of the language of entire words, and thus, it is not as powerful for generating comfort as are the other searching techniques.

> ***Pro-tip:*** Instead of marking in the book, download the puzzle from ***www.feelgreat.duncantooley.com,*** the book extras website, and print several copies. That way you can get the benefit again, if needed, on a fresh puzzle.

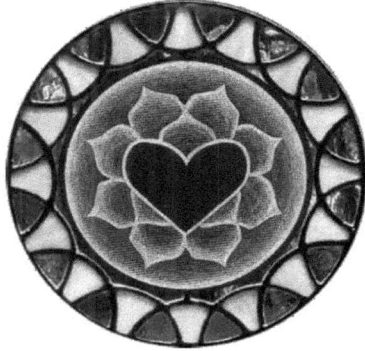

APPENDICES
- RESOURCES FOR THE CURIOUS

- ▶ **A1. Emotional P@#$ Case Study**
- ▶ **A2. Mind-Body-Spirit Model**
- ▶ **A3. Placebo Effect**
- ▶ **A4. Mind Principles**
- ▶ **A5. Interpretation Revelation**
- ▶ **A6. Medical Benefits of Hypnosis**
- ▶ **A7. Hypnosis Myths Busted**

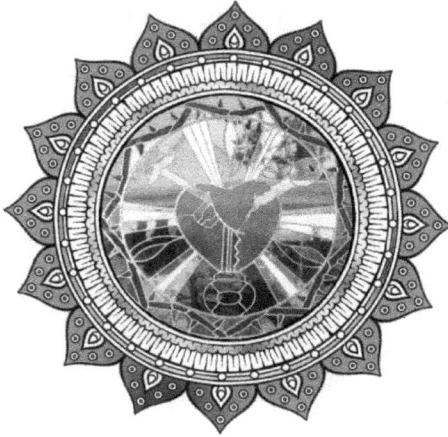

Emotional P@#$ Case Study

Brian, a retired pharmacist, had a nuisance pain with no physical basis that could be identified. Medical tests for stomach issues found nothing organically wrong. His doctor referred him to me in hopes that hypnosis could help him sleep better.

Our first session was difficult. When Brian arrived at my office he seemed confused and needed his wife to help answer my questions. He was very thin, grimaced constantly, and spoke in negatives. He said, "I cannot get to sleep and have been on sleeping pills that barely help. I'm worried all the time about many things but especially about my health. I also have a relentless pain in my stomach that prevents me from eating properly."

The progressive relaxation and hypnotic induction were unsuccessful. He said, "I can't relax or clear my mind of my worries to focus on your instructions."

I asked Brian to breathe deeply as I counted and gently massaged his third eye in a circular motion. He finally relaxed sufficiently to accept affirmations. I gave Brian the motto (that I learned from Winifred Morice), "Every little cell in my body is happy; every little cell in my body is well." I also gave Brian several reminder cards with this same motto imprinted on them to be placed where he would see them frequently during the day. I reminded him, "If you breathe fully when you are in your bed you will relax more." Brian even smiled some as he left our first session.

When I saw Brian the following week, the change in his demeanor was dramatic. He smiled often and was clearly less anxious. He reported no change in the stomach discomfort or in his sleeping pattern. The following is a transcript of our dialog:

Duncan: "What do you think about in bed at night?"

Brian: "Guilt. I was beaten as a child and then I beat my own children and did what I learned from my parents. I have so much remorse and guilt that I hit my children, that I just want to die!"

Duncan: "What do you think will happen when you die?"

Brian: "Eaten up by worms."

Duncan: "What will be eaten up by worms?"

Brian: "My body."

Duncan: "Is that all of you or is there any other part of you?"

Brian: "My soul will go to God."

Duncan: "Where is your guilt? In your body or your soul?"

Brian: (After hesitating) "I guess in my soul."

Duncan: "So dying won't get rid of your guilt, will it?"

Brian: "I guess I'll have to come back again to get rid of it!"

Duncan: "I guess you will have to come back as many times as you need to until you get it right and then you can stay with God?"

Brian: "That makes sense."

Duncan: "So you might as well try to get it right as soon as possible in this life."

Brian: (Nodded an affirmation.)

Duncan: "What good does your guilt serve?"

Brian: "None."

Duncan: "Would you like to get rid of it?"

Brian: "Yes! And the pain in my stomach too!"

When I instructed Brian to relax, he seemed more open to doing so than previously. He loosened his belt to "relieve the pressure on my bloated stomach," as he put it. After a progressive relaxation and hypnotic induction, I led him to imagine descending in an elevator down ten levels to his deepest mind or consciousness.

I told him, "When the elevator doors open you will be greeted by your Higher-Self, that All-Wise, All-Knowing part of you that knows everything about you and wants to help you very much. I will prompt you with questions to ask your Higher-Self. After you ask each question, your Higher-Self will answer with the first thought that comes into your mind. Then say that answer aloud so that I may know it also."

Duncan: "Ask your Higher-Self: 'What is the purpose of the guilt?' Accept the first thought that comes to you;

don't edit or judge it. Just accept it even if you don't understand."

Brian: "Punishment."

Duncan: "Can I speak to that part of Brian that is responsible for the guilt?"

Brian: "Yes."

Duncan: "So you are responsible for the guilt. What is your name?"

Brian: "Brian."

Duncan: "So, Brian, your job is to make Brian feel guilty as a punishment for what he has done. Is that right?"

Brian: "Yes."

Duncan: "Do you like your job?"

Brian: "No."

Duncan: "Would it be alright if you gave up this job and got another job?"

Brian: "Yes."

Duncan: "What other job would you like?"

Brian: "Making Brian comfortable."

Duncan: "Good. So is it acceptable to you to give up making Brian feel guilty, and instead your future job will be to make him feel comfortable?"

Brian: "Yes."

Duncan: "Is this acceptable to all parts of Brian or is there any other part that wants to speak?"

Brian: "Yes; I have something to say. I am Stomach. My job is to keep Brian close to his father."

Duncan "How do you do that?"

Brian: "By hurting."

Duncan: "How does that keep Brian close to his father?"

Brian: "His father's stomach hurt all the time because his wife (Brian's mother) yelled at him all the time."

Duncan: "So you make Brian's stomach hurt all the time because his father's stomach hurt all the time and this is a way for Brian to stay close to his father. Is that right?""

Brian: "Yes."

Duncan: "Do you like this job?"

Brian: "No!"

Duncan: "What job would you rather do instead?"

Brian: "Keep Brian nourished."

Duncan: "Would you be willing to give up the old job if Brian could find a better way to be close to his father?"

Brian: "Yes."

Duncan: "Brian, how would you like to be close to your Father?"

Brian: "He used to kiss me 'Good night' and say 'God bless you!' My mother never kissed me."

Duncan: "Is there some part who will take the job of keeping Brian close to his father by kissing him 'Good night' and saying "God bless you?'"

Brian: "Yes, I will do that!"

Duncan: "What name shall we call this part?"

Brian: "Kiss."

Duncan: "Good, Kiss! Is it acceptable with all the parts of Brian that Stomach will give up hurting and Kiss will remind Brian of his father, and Brian's job is to make Brian comfortable?"

Brian: "Yes."

Duncan: "Are there any other parts of Brian that want to say something?"

Brian: "Yes."

Duncan: "What is your name?"

Brian: "Feet."

Duncan: "Feet, what do you want to say?"

Brian:	"I'm getting numb down here."
Duncan:	"What do you want?"
Brian:	"I want to walk more."
Duncan:	"Brian and all other parts, is that something that you could agree to do?"
Brian:	"Yes, we need the exercise."
Duncan:	"How much and how often will you walk?"
Brian:	"A mile every day."
Duncan:	"Good! Feet, is it acceptable to you that Brian walks a mile every day?"
Brian:	"Yes."
Duncan:	"Is it acceptable to all the parts of Brian that he walk a mile every day?"
Brian:	"Yes."
Duncan:	"Are there any other parts of Brian that have something they want to say?"
Duncan:	(After a few moments of silence). "Good! Brian, thank all your parts for cooperating together."
Duncan:	(After a few moments of silence). "Let all those parts and your Higher-Self fade from your awareness and return your full awareness to the magnificent chamber where the elevator brought you."

I then walked Brian through an imagery process where a column of gentle rain floated down out of the ceiling of this room and mysteriously soaked into the floor. I told Brian that the column of water called out for him to enter into it. He then did enter into the column of water in his imagination.

Duncan:	"It feels like a comfortable warm shower cleansing your body, not only on the outside, but mysteriously on the inside as well. It washes away every damaged cell, every chemical that doesn't belong in your body, every emotion, thought, memory that isn't perfect for you. It feels so good to be cleansed!"

"Look down at your feet to see cloudy water emerging and running off into the ground where it disappears and is soaked down into the earth. The water is flowing out of your body clearer and clearer as your cleansing process completes.

"When the water is completely clear, a magnificent golden light fills you and the entire column. It is a healing, energizing, renewing light that reaches into every corner of your being, restoring everything as good as new, even better than new. It perfects your thoughts, emotions, habits, and body. It tickles you on the inside until you begin to laugh."

"Then you remember the silly rule that someone taught you: Laughing is just the *H* sound on the front of each of the vowels: ha, ha, ha, ha, ha, ha,...... he, he, he, he, he, he, he,... hi, hi, hi, hi, hi, hi, hi,... ho, ho, ho, ho, ho, ho... hu, hu, hu, hu, hu, hu. Isn't that funny?"

I led Brian to repeat affirmations about being comfortable, enjoying life, and every cell being happy and well. He agreed that he would say his motto 20 times each day, that he would concentrate on his breathing as he went to sleep at night, and that he would remember everything that occurred during the session.

Afterward, when I brought Brian back to room awareness, I reviewed his session with him, reminding him of all the key events. He said his stomach still hurt. I reminded him that habits can sometimes take time to change. I encouraged him to say his "Every little cell is happy and well" motto twenty times each day and use the relaxing breathing method upon retiring at night.

When I saw Brian several months later, he reported that his discomfort was totally gone away and that he continued to use his motto in the morning and evening.

Review of the Case Study

Key points to notice for banishing your discomfort:

1. The session started with the progressive relaxation of the *Relaxation Response* process. This was augmented by more relaxation descending in an elevator. The *Relaxation Response* technique is the basis for most health and recovery. Learn to use it habitually.

2. Guided Imagery (visualization, imagination) was used throughout.

3. The interview with Brian's Higher Self is similar to the Talk *to Your Cells* technique (Chapter 1) and asking them what is going on. We all have a connection to the Intelligence that is beyond our conscious mind. When we connect to it, we get amazing truths that we might not otherwise discover.

4. The next section is technically called *parts therapy* in which each of the sub-personalities is interviewed and their role adjusted if needed. (We are all a combination of sub-personalities, and different ones are dominant at different times! Notice how the various parts wanted their voice to be heard and changes made!)

5. The guided imagery of water column and healing light constituted a way to cleanse away the debilitating emotions and reenergize Brian. You can utilize this imagery for yourself. Let your discomfort and any imperfect cells be rinsed away and new, perfect cells be created where there was injury or illness before.

6. The laughing released endorphins and made Brian feel better. Laughing is a discomfort-banishment technique that is available anywhere and anytime.

7. Use concepts from this Case Study in your own journey from discomfort to comfort! Interview your Higher Self, your connection to your spiritual energy, to get answers about what you should do about your discomfort.

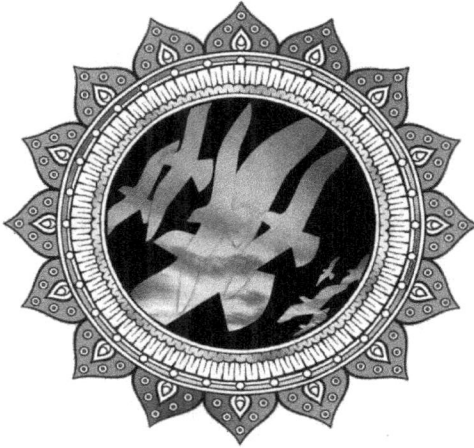

Mind-Body-Spirit Model

What is Mind?

Mind and brain are not the same. We don't understand the role the brain plays in consciousness. We can measure the existence of thoughts (and aspects of consciousness) in the brain, and we can use the predominant frequency of brain waves to determine the level of consciousness. Brain activity of *beta* waves above 13 hertz (cycles per second) indicate high consciousness (alertness, concentration, anticipation). *Alpha* waves from 7 hertz to 13 hertz are associated with tranquil, relaxed wakefulness. This is the brain wave pattern during meditation. *Theta* waves from 4 hertz to 7 hertz are considered the twilight state between sleep and wakefulness. They are associated with hypnosis, dreams, deep meditation, and great creativity. *Delta* waves below-4 hertz are associated with deep dreamless sleep.

What is consciousness? The brain seems to be the physical device for consciousness but not consciousness itself, somewhat like the memory chip in a cell phone or audio music player is the physical device that holds the song, but is not the song. The real gap in our understanding is how consciousness can continue after the organ that is the brain is no longer living. Practically every religion affirms that there is conscious intelligent life after the death of the body. That consciousness must somehow reside beyond the physical limits of the brain.

The common word used to capture this fact is MIND, defined as "That element of a person that enables them to be aware of the world and their experiences, to think, and to feel; the faculty of consciousness and thought."

No one understands everything about how the mind works. Philosophers have speculated for centuries about the mind and consciousness. Scientists believe they are learning more each year, especially since they can monitor activity in certain parts of the brain in real time and relate that to mental activity associated with consciousness. Allusions to consciousness fill poetry, philosophy, religion books, and Shakespeare's plays. Yet consciousness is still a mystery as to how it all works in us. My clients find the "computer model" as an aid to their understanding.

Computer Model of Mind

Computer engineers were very shrewd; they designed computers to be very much like us. When you look at a desktop computer the first thing that you see is the hardware: the screen, keyboard, mouse, printer, and speakers. These are all devices to get the information into or out of the computer. Notice that each of these is connected to the central processing unit, or CPU, with electrical cables. This is like our body with its five senses all connected to our CPU, our brain, by the electrical cables that form our nervous system. Our senses are what get our information into and out of our brain, our central processor.

But what makes the computer really function and do useful work, of course, is the software. There are always two levels of software in every computer. The most obvious level is called the application software. This software is designed to get a specific task accomplished. It is where the works gets done. Typical application software programs are word processor, email, web browser, and spreadsheets. As the size of computers shrank to the size of smart phones, the name of application software shrank to "apps." The apps on your smart phone are today's application software programs on your pocket computer.

Conscience Mind Is Like Application Software

Your conscious mind where you do your work, your rational thought, your analyzing, computation, language, and planning is very much like application software. This is the part of your mind that believes it is in control and makes decisions. It is where you exert willpower. It is that part of your mind that is at this moment pondering these concepts and the implications of the last sentence. It may even be suggesting that you reread three paragraphs for greater understanding!

Underneath the application software in every computer, there is always another level of software that is the operating system. The operating system's role is to make everything work together, handle the many common essential tasks for every application program, and keep the intricacies of program code hidden. The operating system handles the details to keep everything running smoothly so you can do your work without interruption or distraction. Even when your computer seems idle, there are dozens of programs running in the operating system.

Your Subconscious Is Your Operating System

You have an operating system, too. It's your subconscious mind. It runs your body, your reactions, your emotions, and your habits. A habit is like a program stored in your nervous system and controlled by your subconscious. Your interpretation of the signals from your body is a habit program running in your subconscious. This habit generates your awareness of comfort or discomfort.

Your Subconscious Programs

You have thousands of involuntary, automatic, thoughtless responses that take you through your day. When you feel discomfort on a finger from touching a plate that is too hot, you automatically pull your hand back without thinking about it until afterward. Your response was totally automatic; there was no conscious thought involved. These same types of triggered responses apply to thought patterns, emotions, and skills. These are like subroutines, small programs that get you through most of life's activities. Habits are like bigger, more complex programs. Amazing how clever those computer engineers were to design software that works like we do!

Your Subconscious Mind Runs Your Body

Yes, it's true! Your subconscious is controlling your body. Your conscious mind sometimes controls your skeletal muscles, as when you decide to stretch. If you consciously think about it, you can also control your breathing and your blinking; but if you don't think about these, they will continue without your conscious thought.

All the rest of your body's *automatic* processes, like blood pumping and oxygenation, digestion, wound healing, cell regeneration, waste collection, immune responses, and hundreds more, are not under your conscious control. They are under the control of your personal operating system, your subconscious mind. The medical profession calls this your autonomic nervous system. The neurons in the autonomic nervous system attach to your organs, and like the brain, are the physical support for the metaphysical activity of the mind that continues to keep your life force active within your body.

What does this computer program analogy mean for relief of your discomfort? It means that your goal becomes having one or more relief techniques for nuisance discomfort running automatically as a habit. The relief method is like a program upgrade for your subconscious. When you install your upgrade, you will have obtained relief without drugs. You will have trained your brain to feel great, perhaps without your conscious mind even noticing the program change!

Energy Source

Electricity from a battery or connection to the power grid is what powers a computer. What powers you? Stop reading for a few moments and consider how you answer this question. What powers you? How you answer this question depends on your culture, education, religious background, and life experiences. Whatever your answer, it is important because it is ultimately your source of power for overcoming the discomfort that you experience. Some call it soul or life-force or Spirit. What do YOU call your ultimate source of life energy?

Connectivity

A computer also needs a connection to other resources for software updates and information. That connectivity is through the Internet to all the resources on the worldwide web. That Internet connectivity also provides connectivity to other individuals via email, teleconferences, or interactive video. This connectivity is essential for modern computers, including mobile devices.

Connectivity to others and to resources has always been part of life, but because of technology, the flow is more obvious with our smart-phone in our hand frequently throughout the day. What is your connectivity for operating system upgrades, access to remote resources, communication with remote individuals, or even deceased loved ones? Some call it intuition; others admit to some psychic powers. What do you call YOUR connections?

The popular name for connectivity to the resources of all living things and metaphysical energy is the *Super-conscious mind*. It is what powers you, no matter what your belief system. It gives you life by connecting you to all other life in the universe, to all resources past, present, and future (timeless), and to the divine. Your super-conscious mind is your discomfort-relief connection to your life source and to the resources beyond the material.

Many call these two components of energizing life-force and connectivity by the term *spirit*. Therefore, it is common to speak of us humans as composed of body, mind, and spirit, just as your computer is composed of hardware, software, electricity, and network connection.

You are a complete being integrating Mind, Body, and Spirit. Your goal to end discomfort and feel great will include techniques that encompass each of these aspects of your being.

Hidden Auto-Programs

Your subconscious mind is the home for your habits. A habit is like a program stored in your nervous system and controlled by your subconscious. You love habits because they free your conscious mind. You send a repetitive activity down to your subconscious as a program (habit) that you can run whenever you need without requiring conscious thought or energy.

Tying Your Shoes

When you first learned how to tie your shoes, it took conscious concentration to learn the pattern and teach your finger muscles the routine. As you repeated it, it got easier and easier. Once you repeated it enough, it became a habit. What that means is that you sent the conscious pattern of finger movements down to your subconscious as a fixed program to be run anytime you needed it. All you have to do now is put on shoes with laces, and the next thing you know, they are tied without any conscious thought. Your *shoe-lace-tying* program was automatically invoked to automatically fire your neurons to move your fingers in the right pattern to execute the tied knot. Meanwhile, your conscious mind could have been thinking about anything, but most likely was thinking about where you were about to walk once your shoes were tied.

Walking

The same is true for walking. As an infant, you spent conscious energy over an extended period of time learning how to walk. You concentrated on firing neurons to move muscles in a coordinated pattern that imitated what you saw adults doing. You worked hard at it because you wanted to be able to move around as easily as you saw adults doing. Their encouragement motivated you to keep trying to get the pattern right even though you kept falling.

Finally you figured it out and wobbled your first steps. With more practice, your walking got smoother, but still required conscious effort. Then, eventually, it required less and less conscious thought as it became a routine program or habit.

Now everything about walking is so ingrained into your subconscious that it no longer requires conscious thought. Once you decide (with your conscious mind) that you want to walk some place, Your subconscious autopilot uses your stored program *walking* to handle all of the details of the right muscles to move at the right times. (Note: Walking is an exceedingly complex program incorporating feedback from the feet that influences the formulation of the next commands to move the leg and foot muscles. That complexity has hindered the development of *walking* robots).

Driving

Driving is probably the most complex physical habit that you have developed. When you first learned how to drive, it was difficult to simultaneously focus on all those details to do at the same time. Now they do not require conscious thought.

When the brake lights of the car in front of you light up, your foot automatically comes off the accelerator and onto the brake pedal without conscious thought. When you want to turn, you involuntarily turn on the turn signal. These, and many other actions, are now all part of the automatic habit-program you call *driving.*

You have probably experienced, more than once, arriving at your destination and not remembering any details of the trip. That's because your conscious mind was busy with other things while your subconscious drove the car for the entire trip, taking care of all the details automatically.

Pavlov

Ivan Pavlov was a Russian scientist who won the 1904 Nobel Prize in Physiology/Medicine for his research on the digestive system and involuntary reflex actions. Pavlov is most famous for his experiment of ringing a bell when he fed his dogs. After doing this for several days, he rang the bell without putting any food out. His dogs salivated at the sound of the bell. He did it again and again. They salivated again and again, even though there was no food.

This behavior pattern has come to be known as a *conditioned reflex.* You can also call it a *subconscious program*, or an *automatic reaction,* or a *thoughtless response.* In the dogs' experience databases, food and salivating were connected to the bell ringing. The ringing bell sound accessed the bell-ringing memory in the dogs' databases and activated the associated responses. Pavlov also studied involuntary reactions to stress and discomfort.

These conditioned reflexes from the database of prior experiences work similarly in humans. That means emotions and sensations of discomfort, grief, anger, sadness, or joy associated with prior experiences are automatically triggered by similar new circumstances in each of us; that means in me and in you! They are a type of habit.

Why is this illustration of habits, automatic subconscious programs, and conditioned reflexes, important? Its purpose is to help you grasp the very essential truth: your subconscious is running most of your life. Your conscious mind likes to think that it is in control. However, just like in your computer, there are many programs running in your operating system, in your subconscious, about which you are not aware. You can add more habits that will similarly perform automatically. Let relief be such a habit!

Make Your Relief Techniques a Habit

The impact of this for your comfort level is that your current interpretation of discomfort is running as a subconscious program, a habitual way of interpreting bodily sensations. The goal for your feel-great project is to have one or more relief techniques running automatically as a habit program for any nuisance discomfort. Then you will have converted discomfort to comfort without drugs by the power of your mind. (And perhaps it will have been so easy and automatic that you did not even notice!)

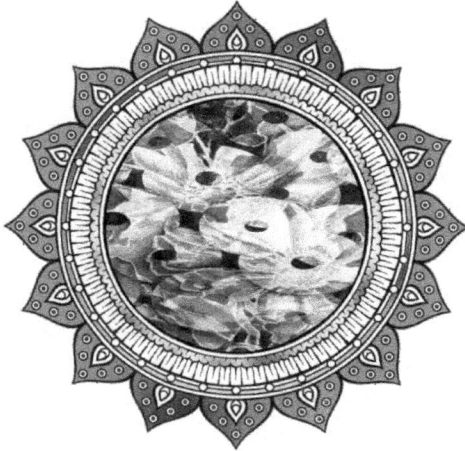

Placebo Effect

The Power of Belief

The *Placebo Effect* (also called the placebo response) is the phenomenon in which a person experiences a beneficial medical effect unexplainably resulting from an inactive substance such as sugar, distilled water, or saline solution. Usually the person either believes that the substance is a remedial medicine, or that it could be (as in an informed clinical trial). However, improvement can occur even if the person knows that it is a fake, not a real medical remedy.

How does this happen? Western medical science has no answer, but by now you know that your mind is running your body. Therefore you know that if you believe that a substance is curative, it will have beneficial effects. Even if the substance is not certainly curative, but may be, as in a blind trial, the hope and anticipation can have a curative effect. Even in the case where you know that this is just a placebo, the language associations around the word *placebo* conjure imaginings of cure, and hence have a positive effect.

The placebo effect is very real. It is an inconvenience and annoyance to physicians and pharmaceutical companies because it ruins any simple mechanistic view of illnesses and what must be done to remedy symptoms. Typical blind clinical trials for new drug therapies have as their first objective that those taking the drug improve at least as much as those who took the placebo instead of the drug. Often all it takes for a new drug to get to market is a very small percentage symptom improvement beyond the improvement in those trial participants who received only the placebo. In expensive, highly controlled drug trials, the placebo effect usually results in improvements in the range of 30% upwards to over 50% improvement.

Your Placebo

Why is this important for your ending of discomfort? It proves the power of your mind over your body and over discomfort. From all the fuss in the pharmaceutical industry and by the FDA over the placebo effect, you know that it is real! YOU can exercise the placebo effect for yourself to feel better. You don't need a fake pill to relieve your discomfort because you know that you can imagine taking the fake pill and believe that it will work, and it will! (You can even skip thinking about the fake pill and just tell yourself to get better!)

Without specifically invoking the placebo effect by name, the effect is certainly at work in many of the techniques presented in this book. A more generalized statement of the placebo effect is *"belief leads to beneficial change without any identifiable tangible cause."*

Study: The placebo effect works not only with medications, but also with other remedies, even for surgery, as exemplified by this study: "A Controlled Trial of Arthroscopic Surgery for Osteoarthritis of the Knee" (*New England Journal of Medicine*, July 11, 2002, Vol. 347 No. 2)

BACKGROUND: Many patients report symptomatic relief after having arthroscopy (use of tiny fiber optic camera inserted into knee) for osteoarthritis, but it is unclear how the procedure achieves this result. To evaluate the efficacy of arthroscopy for osteoarthritis of the knee, a randomized, placebo-controlled trial was done.

METHOD: 180 patients with osteoarthritis of the knee were randomly assigned to receive arthroscopic debridement (removal of the damaged tissue), arthroscopic lavage (therapeutic rinsing), or placebo surgery. Patients in the placebo group received skin incisions and underwent a simulated debridement without insertion of the arthroscope. Patients and assessors were blinded to group assignment. Outcomes were assessed over a 24-month period with the use of five self-reported scores: 3 for pain, 2 for function, and an objective walking and stair climbing test. The trial was completed by165 patients.

RESULTS: At no point did either of the intervention groups report less discomfort or better function than the placebo group.

CONCLUSIONS: In this controlled trial involving patients with osteoarthritis of the knee, the outcomes after arthroscopic lavage or arthroscopic debridement were no better than those after a placebo procedure.

In other words, BELIEVING they had the healing surgery was just as effective as having it! That's the PLACEBO EFFECT of your mind!

What conclusion do you draw from this? Exercise the placebo effect for yourself by believing you have the power to dispel your discomfort and feel great. Then it will happen! It will happen not only because of the placebo effect, but also because you really do have this power! The placebo effect is witness to the power of your mind.

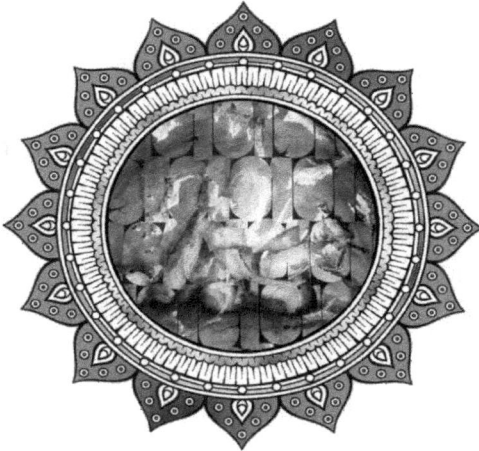

Mind Principles

How Your Mind Works

These principles of how the mind works are fundamental to the mind-over-body discomfort-relieving techniques in this book and the basis of my coaching. These formulations are from the teachings of Shelley Stockwell-Nicholas, PhD:

- You create your reality by your thoughts.
- You accept suggestions best in the language of your dominant sense.

- Your Self-Talk is hypnotizing you into a belief which affects everything.
- Thoughts are real things that radiate energy to affect people, events, and circumstances.
- Your mind affects your body and your body affects your mind.
- You remember and react best when strong emotion is attached.
- You imitate what you see your role models do.
- Change only occurs at the subconscious level.
- Change only occurs in the present moment.
- Readiness for change is half the change.
- You are single-minded. (You can only hold one thing in your mind at a time.)
- Habits run your life.
- What you affirm, you create.
- What you resist, you reinforce.
- What you insist, you resist.
- Your thoughts of anticipation initiate, create, and exaggerate.
- Energy flows where attention goes.
- Once you accept a belief, you find and emphasize what supports it, and you discount or ignore what contradicts your belief.
- You seek pleasure and avoid (or ignore) discomfort.
- *Try* implies failure. The harder you try, the more difficult it becomes.
- Imagination is more important than knowledge or logic.
- Your subconscious connects to the super-conscious Source of Ultimate Wisdom.

- Strong words work best.

- Your subconscious mind is literal. Use simple clear words and phrases.

- Repetition reinforces. Repetition plus repetition reinforces more than double.

Your mind is working all the time as the most complex machine in creation. The above is a short list of principles that describe some of the features of your mind that have been discovered. Apply these principles to help you discover the additional principles that are already working in your mind.

Pro-Tip: Understanding these principles and making them part of your belief system and actions will ease discomfort and promote feeling great. They will have a subtle, powerful effect on your entire life! A good approach is to take one principle at a time and turn it into a question about how it applies to you.

For example, based on the first three principles above:

- What reality am I creating in my life by my dominant thoughts?

- What is my strongest or dominant sense? Am I mostly visual, or do I learn and express through sounds, or smells, or feelings?

- What belief that isn't working for me is coming from my Self-Talk?

Ask the question(s) to yourself just before falling asleep and let your subconscious work on the answer while you sleep. You will awaken with more clarity. You may even dream about your question. Ask a different question each night, (unless your intuition suggests a repetition).

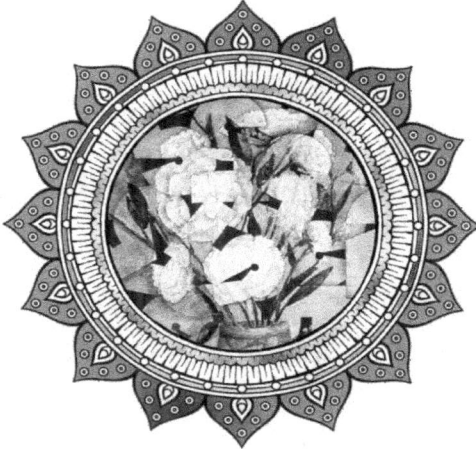

Interpretation Revelation

P@#$ Is an Interpretation

When something happens in your body, your brain applies meaning and triggers emotion to interpret what is going on. Without your brain's interpretation, there would be no p@#$! Furthermore, your brain can interpret p@#$ when it should not!

In 2002, I had the startling revelation that discomfort is an interpretation and not something real in itself. I experienced the following hands-on scientific demonstration exhibit at the San Francisco Exploratorium:

Two coils of small copper tubing are positioned so that they partially overlap and are intertwined only in the center. Cool water is circulated through one coil and warm water is circulated through the other coil.

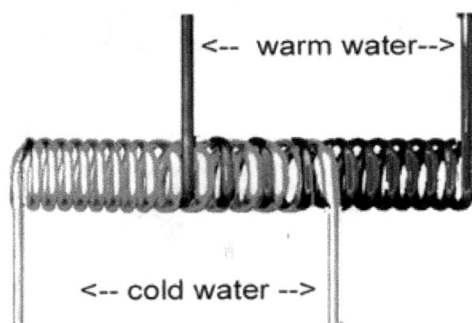

When I followed the exhibit instructions to place my hands on the outer ends of the coils, I experienced a cool sensation on one hand and a warm sensation on my other hand, as I expected.

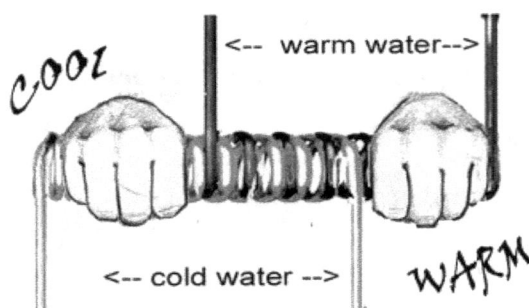

When I followed the next instruction, the unimaginable occurred! When I placed both hands around the center section where the cold and warm coils were intertwined, I was startled to experience intense p@#$ in my hands!

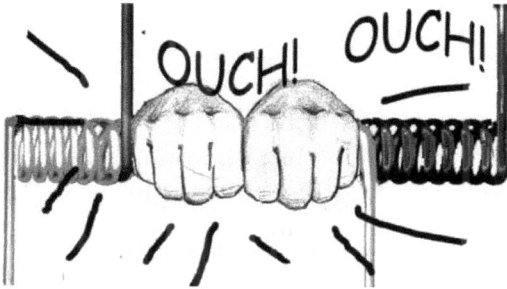

Huh? What is this p@#$ all about? It is only the same cool and warm water! The answer comes from how we process (interpret) information from our senses.

Sensory Input to Interpretation

To grasp how this interpretation process works, imagine for a moment (or perhaps remember when it already happened to you!) the following scenario:

While driving on the multi-lane highway in heavy traffic (that means cars in the lanes on both sides of you), you see a black object in your lane in the road ahead. You have to make a quick decision about whether to run over it or slam on your brakes and risk being hit from behind. Immediately, you automatically (in milliseconds) begin to match the color, texture, shape and size of this object against your database of previous experiences with road debris and black objects. Is it shiny like a plastic trash bag? Is the shape like that of a piece of tire? Does it have sharp edges like a piece of metal or soft edges like an animal? Within fractions of a second, you decide on the best match and decide what action to take.

The longer you live, and the more highway driving you do, the richer becomes your database of previous experiences to predict the best response for each of life's highway driving challenges.

Database Search Fail

But what happens if your database of previous experiences does not contain a match for your current sensory input? That is what happened to me with the cool and warm coils at the Exploratorium exhibit! I had never sensed anything with cool and warm bands adjacent to each other on the palms of my hands. Therefore, my brain's database search for interpretation came up empty-handed. My brain has a default program about what to do in that case to get me out of danger: it interpreted this situation as dangerous and triggered my brain's *pain center.* That signal caused me to feel pain, and more importantly for my safety, to let go of the coils!

In this case my brain's interpretation was incorrect. There was no danger and no need to send a discomfort signal to cause me to let go. There was no difference in the external stimuli and no difference in what my skin felt between my first hand placement (with a single temperature on each hand) and the center hand placement (with mixed temperatures). What was different was the signal processing in my brain that placed a painful interpretation on the event!

Other people had the same reaction that I did. The purpose of the exhibit was to show how pain is not always deserved. The best definition of *P@#$* is *an interpretation of something perceived to be happening in the body.* This has a profound implication: If it is an *interpretation,* just change your interpretation! YES, you absolutely can do it!

> *The REIGN of PAIN is mainly in the BRAIN —*
> *and your MIND is the THRONE*
> *from which the KING REIGNS.*
>
> --Duncan Tooley

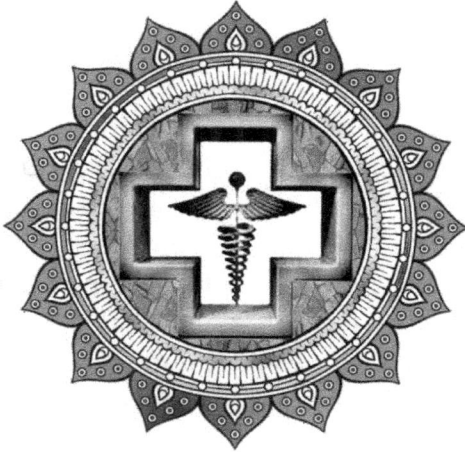

Medical Benefits of Hypnosis

Your subconscious mind runs your body. Therefore it follows that it should be possible to effect biological changes in your body by giving your subconscious mind instructions through hypnosis. Thousands of medical studies verify the truth of this logical conclusion.

Below is a partial list of the medical issues that benefit from hypnosis. Following the list is the abstract of each study that validated the hypnosis benefits.

Medical Issues Benefitting from Hypnosis-(partial list)

Acne
Addiction
Allergy
Alcoholism
Anesthesia for pain
Anesthesia for surgery
Asthma
Auto-immune disorders
Back pain (chronic)
Bleeding (surgery)
Boils (furuncles)
Breast cancer surgery
Cardiac surgery
Chemotherapy side effects
Childbirth
Constipation (chronic)
Dementia
Dermatitis
Eczema (neurodermatitis)
Face skin redness (rosacea)
Fibromyalgia
Hair loss (alopecia)
Hair pulling (trichotillomania)
Headaches (chronic)
Healing from injury
Healing from surgery
Hemophilia
Herpes

Hives (urticaria)
Hypertension
Impotence
Insomnia
Irritable bowel syndrome
Itching (pruritus)
Mouth-burning (glossodynia)
Neuralgia
Pain suppression
Panic attacks
Peptic ulcers
Phobias
Psoriasis
Psychogenic weakness
Seborrhea
Sedation (for surgery)
Skin - dry/scaly (ichthyosis)
Skin color loss (vitiligo)
Skin discoloration
Smoking cessation
Surgery recovery (all types)
Sweating excess (hyperhidrosis)
Thyroidectomies
Tinnitus (ringing in ears)
Urinary incontinence
Warts (verruca vulgaris)
Weight loss
Wound healing

Extra: Print this *Medical Issues Benefitting from Hypnosis* from the book extras website:
www.feelgreat.duncantooley.com

The Validating Studies

Documented Results in Contemporary Medicine

A review study of over a hundred clinical studies of hypnosis for medical procedures documents that hypnosis is beneficial for allergy, anesthesia for pain, anesthesia for surgery, warts, dermatitis, irritable bowel syndrome, peptic ulcers, abdominal surgery, healing from injury or surgery, hemophilia, hypertension, headaches, childbirth, asthma, smoking cessation, fibromyalgia, impotence, and urinary incontinence. *"Many important trials reviewed have helped to establish the role of hypnosis in contemporary medicine. These trials have established the utility and efficacy of hypnosis for several medical conditions, either alone or as part of the treatment regimen."* (Cf. References, Study 13)

Success Rate 77 Percent for Drug Addiction

In a measure of 18 clients (15 for alcoholism or alcohol abuse, 2 cocaine addiction, and 1 for marijuana addiction), hypnosis showed a 77 percent success rate for at least a 1-year follow-up. (Cf. References, Study 14)

Hypnotherapy Bests Psychotherapy for Addicts.

In a comparative study of hypnotherapy and psychotherapy in the treatment of methadone addicts, significantly more methadone addicts quit with hypnosis. At six month follow up, 94% percent of the subjects who received hypnosis remained narcotic free. (Cf. References, Study 15)

Lost More Weight than 90% of Others & Kept It Off

Researchers analyzed 18 studies comparing a cognitive behavioral therapy such as relaxation training, guided imagery, self-monitoring, or goal setting with the same therapy supplemented by hypnosis. Those who received the hypnosis lost more weight than 90 percent of those not receiving hypnosis and maintained the weight loss two years after treatment ended. (Cf. References, Study 16)

Most Effective Way to Stop Smoking

Hypnosis is the most effective way of giving up smoking, according to the largest ever scientific comparison of ways of breaking the habit. A meta-analysis, statistically combining results of more than 600 studies of 72,000 people from America and Europe to compare various methods of quitting. On average, hypnosis was over three times as effective as nicotine replacement methods and 15 times as effective as trying to quit alone. (Cf. References, Study 17)

Guided Imagery Improves Cardiac Surgery Results

"Cardiac surgery patients who listened to a preoperative guided imagery surgical tape had significantly less pain, anxiety and two days shorter hospital stay." (Cf. References, Study 18)

Hypnosis Beneficial for Breast Cancer Surgeries

In a randomized study of 200 women undergoing surgery for breast cancer, those who received a brief hypnosis session before entering the operating room required less anesthesia and pain medication during surgery, and reported less pain, nausea, fatigue, and discomfort after surgery than women who did not receive hypnosis. The overall cost of surgery was also significantly less for women undergoing hypnosis. (Cf. References, Study 19)

Blood Flow Control during Surgery

In a trial with 93 spinal surgery patients at the University of California (Davis) Medical Center, those who received specific instructions about blood flow lost about half as much blood compared to the controls and a third group taught relaxation techniques. (Cf. References, Study 1)

Hypnosis Re-routes Signal Away from Pain Center

When hot plates were applied to volunteers, substantial pain was induced, and the live brain scan showed the signal routed to the pain center. Under hypnosis little or no pain was experienced and the brain scans revealed that the signal was routed to other parts of the brain, and not the pain center. *"It helps to dispel prejudice about hypnosis as a technique to manage pain because we can show an objective, measurable change in brain activity linked to a reduced perception of pain."* (Cf. References, Study 20)

Hypnosis Benefits Fibromyalgia

"In a controlled study, 40 patients with refractory fibromyalgia were randomly allocated to treatment with either hypnotherapy or physical therapy for 12 weeks with follow up at 24 weeks. Compared with the patients in the physical therapy group, the patients in the hypnotherapy group showed a significantly better outcome." (Cf. References, Study 21)

Hypnosis Improves or Cures Dermatologic Disorders

A comprehensive review of dermatology studies spanning 32 years that involved hypnosis concluded: *"A wide spectrum of dermatologic disorders may be improved or cured using hypnosis as an alternative or complementary therapy, including acne excoriee, alopecia areata, atopic dermatitis, congenital ichthyosiform erythroderma, dyshidrotic dermatitis, erythromelalgia, furuncles, glossodynia, herpes simplex, hyperhidrosis, ichthyosis vulgaris, lichen planus, neurodermatitis, nummular dermatitis, postherpetic neuralgia, pruritus, psoriasis, rosacea, trichotillomania, urticaria, verruca vulgaris, and vitiligo."* (Cf. References, Study 22)

Hypnosis Effective for Irritable Bowel Syndrome

"Previous research from the United Kingdom has shown hypnotherapy to be effective in the treatment of irritable bowel syndrome (IBS). The current study provides a systematic replication of this work in the United States." (Cf. References, Study 23)

Preoperative Suggestions Improve Abdominal Surgery Outcomes.

In a single-blind trial of abdominal surgery patients, to whom a 5 minute script was read preoperatively suggesting increased gastrointestinal motility after surgery, the suggestion group had significantly shorter ileus time (disruption of bowel movement) and was discharged two days earlier, with an estimated savings of $1200 (1993 dollars, Cf. References, Study 24)

Hypnosis for Dementia

Forensic psychologist, Dr. Simon Duff, (Univ. of Liverpool) compared the effects of hypnosis therapy with those of mainstream therapies for people suffering from dementia, and group therapy in which participants were encouraged to discuss news and current affairs. Working in partnership with Dr. Dan Nightingale over a 9-month period, Duff established that people living with dementia who had been given hypnosis therapy exhibited improved concentration, memory and socialization compared to the other two treatment groups. Relaxation, motivation and daily living activities also improved with the use of hypnosis. (Cf. References, Study 25)

Hypnosis Speeds Wound Healing

In a randomized, controlled trial, 18 healthy women were randomized to one of the three treatments after breast reduction surgery: usual care, additional supportive attention, or additional hypnosis sessions targeting accelerated wound healing. The hypnosis group's objectively observed wound healing (digital imagery and staff blind to groups) was significantly greater than the other two groups, indicating that use of a targeted hypnotic intervention can accelerate postoperative wound healing. (Cf. References, Study 26)

Hypnosis Speeds Fracture Repair

In a study at Mass. General's Dept. of Bone and Joint Disease in Boston, 12 adults with bone fractures were followed for 12 weeks, to measure how hypnosis accelerated their healing. Radiographic results showed dramatically improved healing at 6 weeks in the hypnosis patients. Orthopedic assessments of mobility, strength and need for analgesics showed greater improvement in the hypnosis patients at weeks 1, 3 and 9. The hypnotic intervention included audio taped suggestions to reduce swelling, stimulate tissue growth, and fusion at the injury site, and counteract pain and stress; and imagery rehearsals of greater mobility, enhanced bone strength and recovery of normal activities. (Cf. References, Study 27)

Hypnosis for Burns

"Hypnosis has a part to play in nearly every aspect of burn care, from the initial visit through tubbing and grafting, and finally to rehabilitation. Early hypnosis attenuates the inflammatory response to the injury, limiting the usual progression of the burn from first degree to second degree, or from second to third. Procedural pain can be controlled. Guilt or anger about the accident need to be alleviated, caloric intake can be increased, and active participation in physical therapy can be enhanced." (Cf. References, Study 28)

Hypnosis and Female Incontinence

Fifty incontinent women with proved detrusor instability completed 12 sessions of hypnosis (symptom removal by direct suggestion and "ego strengthening") over one month.

At the end of the 12 sessions, 29 patients were entirely symptom free, 14 improved, and 7 unchanged. Three months later, cystometry in 44 of the patients showed conversion of the cystometrogram to stability in 22 and a significant improvement in a further 16; only 6 showed no objective improvement. ..."*It is concluded that psychological factors are very important in "idiopathic" detrusor instability and that hypnotherapy is effective for incontinence due to this disorder.*" (Cf. References, Study 29)

Hypnosis and Male Sexual Dysfunction

A study comprised 79 men in whom clinical and laboratory examinations revealed no organic cause for their impotence were treated with testosterone (20 men), trazodone (21 men), hypnosis (20 men), or a placebo (18 men), all of comparable age groupings. Their reported results by interview at 4, 6 and 8 weeks after treatment were verified by interviewing their partners. Conclusion: *"The only treatment superior to placebo seemed to be hypnosis."* (Cf. References, Study 30)

Medical Hypnosis Underutilized

Five case histories demonstrate the dramatic and sometimes unexpected beneficial outcomes of medical hypnosis. *"Hypnosis is suitable for patients with the following medical conditions: chronic headache, chronic back pain, psychogenic weakness or paralysis, chronic constipation, irritable bowel syndrome, panic attacks and phobias."* (Cf. References, Study 31)

Hypnosis Works as General Anesthesia

197 thyroidectomies and 21 cervical explorations for hyperparathyroidism were performed under hypno-sedation and compared to a closely matched population of patients operated on under general anesthesia. All patients having hypno-sedation reported a very pleasant experience, had significantly less postoperative pain, significantly reduced analgesic use, significantly shorter

hospital stay, providing a substantial reduction of the medical care costs. Their postoperative convalescence was significantly improved, and full return to social or professional activity was significantly shortened. (Cf. References, Study 32)

Hypnosis Makes Tinnitus Nuisance into Pleasure

A combination of relaxation and imagery was used to teach an altered perception of their chronic tinnitus to a series of clients, for all of whom medical intervention had proved ineffective. After some training sessions, the hum which had been troubling them became a cue for relaxation and peace. Thus, whenever they became aware of their tinnitus it came to be welcomed where prior to intervention it had been a constant irritant. (Cf. References, Study 33)

Hypnosis Permits Ignoring Tinnitus Noise

32 patients, variously diagnosed as suffering from tinnitus, were treated with hypnosis. Treatment consisted of a 1-hour consultation with the physician followed by 4 weeks of daily home practice while listening to an audio-tape recording of approximately 15 minutes duration. 22 of the patients treated learned in only 1 month to disregard the disturbing noise. (Cf. References, Study 34)

Mind-Body Hypnotic Imagery in the Treatment of Auto-Immune Disorders

A systematic review of the literature on the connection between the brain and the immune system and its clinical implications. It then provides a rational foundation for the role of using hypnosis and imagery to therapeutically influence the immune system. Five case examples are provided with illustrated instructions for clinicians on how hypnosis and imagery may be utilized in the treatment of patients with auto-immune disorders. (Cf. References, Study 36)

Hypnosis: An Alternate Approach to Insomnia

"Insomnia sleep disorders can be divided into primary and secondary types. Primary sleep disorders have an autonomous function in the central nervous system. Secondary sleep disorders can result from causes such as depression, pain, anxiety, lifestyle change, etc. Hypnosis seems to be most effective in dealing with the problems of a secondary nature." (Cf. References, Study 37).

Hypnosis for Nausea and Vomiting in Cancer Chemotherapy

Six randomized controlled trials that evaluated the effectiveness of hypnosis in chemotherapy-induced nausea and vomiting (CINV) were analyzed. The clinical commentaries reported a large positive effect, including statistically significant reductions in anticipatory and CINV. (Cf. References, Study 38)

Other Hypnosis Medical Studies

There are thousands of studies of the medical benefits of hypnosis. The above list is just a sampling for the some of the most common medical issues. If you did not find your medical issue listed above, do your own internet search by typing into a search engine such as Google "medical study of hypnosis for ...(your issue)."

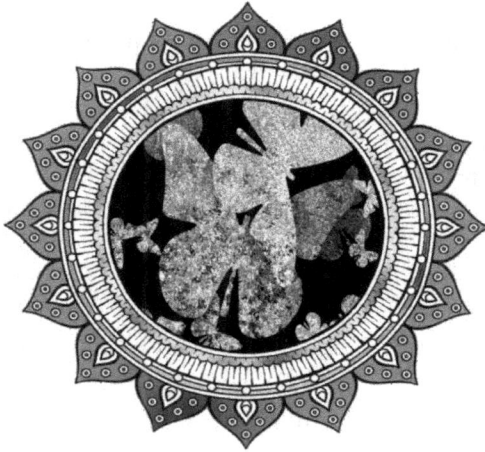

Hypnosis Myths Busted

The Truth in the 11 Worst Hypnosis Myths

There is a saying that every myth has an element of truth in it. Hypnosis is still surrounded by myths in popular culture, and that saying applies to these, my favorites as the worst hypnosis myths. Here are the 11 worst hypnosis myths with the element of *truth* on which they are based, and the *facts* about those myths that bust them.

Myth #1:
Hypnosis is associated with magic, the supernatural, or the work of the devil.

Basis #1: Results of hypnosis appear magical. (My client who came to quit smoking proclaimed this on his second visit: "It's like magic! I haven't had or wanted a cigarette since our session. I don't understand it! How can it be that I am no longer interested in cigarettes?")

Basis #2: Results of hypnosis cannot be adequately explained. What we cannot totally explain by science is often considered *beyond the natural laws* as we understand them, or *supernatural.* (Remember that Galileo Galilei was condemned of heresy by the Inquisition in 1615 for stating that the earth is not at the center of the universe and that it moves around the sun).

Basis #3: Whatever is not understood is often regarded as evil.

Fact: Hypnosis is a natural human state experienced by everyone. It has been extensively studied scientifically. Although we still don't understand much about the mind, we do know how to focus its powers to get results through hypnosis. Hypnotherapy is based on many years of clinical research and documentation by famous psychologists.

Fact: Hypnosis was approved for medical and dental use by the British Medical Association in 1955, by the Pope in 1956, by the American Medical Association in 1958, and endorsed by the American Psychological Association in 1960. Hypnosis is now used in many hospitals. (Hospitals often give hypnosis another name, like visualization or guided imagery, to sidestep this myth).

Myth #2:
A hypnotist is a person who has mysterious or unusual magic-like powers.

Basis: What we don't understand appears magic-like to us.

Fact: A hypnotist does not possess any unusual powers. Hypnotherapists are not psychics, magicians, palm-readers, and do not claim any "special powers." The hypnotist has learned the science and art of effective communication with the subconscious.

Fact: Hypnotists know that everyone hypnotizes themselves and that the trance state is a normal part of everyday life. You are entranced by music, by love, by art, by yoga, in meditation, in prayer, and in the boredom of freeway driving. The hypnotist assists you to return to a trance state where you communicate more directly with your inner wisdom to make your desired change.

Fact: Anyone can learn the skills and become a certified hypnotherapist with the proper training. The hypnotist may teach people how to hypnotize themselves whenever they want, as we routinely do at Tooley Hypnosis.

Myth #3:

Hypnosis means being put to sleep or into unconsciousness. It means a loss of control and being *out!*

Basis: Whenever we see a person being very still with their eyes closed, we think they are either asleep or unconscious, and hopefully not dead!

Fact: In hypnosis you are awake in an active state of heightened inner awareness where you can communicate with the hypnotist and continue to make choices and decisions. It is an opportunity to have a conversation with your Higher Self. Because you are so inwardly focused, you relax your muscles with closed eyes and your body is motionless. Therefore, if people see you, they might think that you were asleep or unconscious because that is usually the case when we see someone still with their eyes closed.

Fact: Sometimes a hypnotized person appears to go to sleep. When this happens it is because the person is completely relaxed and wanted or needed to sleep. They still take on the hypnotic suggestions.

Fact: Listening to a hypnosis audio recording at bedtime is a wonderful way to both reinforce your desired change and relax comfortably into sleep. I recommend it. Your subconscious is most receptive as you fall asleep or sleep. See the first or last page of this book for information about hypnosis recordings.

Myth #4:
The hypnotist will be able to control my mind.

Basis #1: In entertainment hypnosis, the volunteers do what the hypnotist instructs, even if it is silly or something they would not ordinarily do.

Basis #2: Mind control continues to be a popular and profitable science fiction theme for entertainment media.

Fact: No one can control your mind, unless you let them (or unless it's your mother!) Your hypnotherapist gives you suggestions that you want based on the information you provide during the interview. You remain free to decide to follow a suggestion or not, whatever you choose.

Myth #5:
I will embarrass myself by revealing something I have kept secret. Hypnosis can get someone to confess.

Basis: "The silly actions of volunteers in entertainment hypnosis seem embarrassing. If they do those embarrassing things under hypnosis, maybe I will too!"

Fact: Hypnosis for therapy is not hypnosis for entertainment. You will only speak about what is necessary to resolve the issue that you have chosen for hypnosis resolution. Your therapist doesn't care what you may have done, and furthermore, is bound to keep it confidential. Your hypnotherapist is only there to help you achieve what you want, and has probably heard it all before anyway. With hypnosis, you can resolve an issue by admitting to yourself its source without telling the details to the hypnotist. The hypnotist's role is to hold a mirror so that you can see yourself (and your own inner wisdom) more clearly.

Myth #6:
A person in a hypnotic state may not be easily awakened and may remain in that state for a long time. Hypnosis is a dangerous experience.

Basis: Speculation that a hypnotized person is in a very deep, comatose state and that the action of a hypnotist is necessary to bring a person out of that state.

Fact: Awakened is not the proper term, because the person was never asleep. The hypnotist knows and uses the correct method to bring a person back from a trance state to *normal room awareness* at the end of the session. Even if this were not done, the hypnotized person will exit the hypnosis state naturally when ready.

Fact: There is no historical record of anyone ever failing to emerge from a hypnotic state!

Fact: As part of your self-hypnosis training, you will learn both how to put yourself into a trance and how to bring yourself out of a trance whenever you want. Hypnosis is very safe and is in fact, a state of hyper-awareness. My clients report hearing every little sound, but are able to ignore them. If there were an emergency, you would be able to come out of the hypnotic state naturally by opening your eyes and stretching or speaking.

Myth #7:

I can't be hypnotized because my mind is too strong and disciplined.

Basis: Some people report that they tried hypnosis and they were not hypnotized.

Fact: Because hypnosis is such a natural, familiar state, many people who are successfully hypnotized do not think they were hypnotized until they experience the results that they programmed themselves to achieve under hypnosis. Many of my clients tell me later that they didn't think anything happened until they experienced their desired change in their life.

Fact: Because hypnosis accomplishes change in the subconscious without active participation of the conscious mind, the conscious mind afterward is often unaware of the changes as they take place. I have had clients who did not notice that their life had dramatically changed because it felt so familiar, natural, and effortless. They became aware that what they had programmed under hypnosis was now occurring in their life only when a friend or family member called their attention to their changed behavior. Conscious willpower was not required because their subconscious easily implemented their desired adjustment.

Fact: There is a spectrum of ease of going into hypnosis. Some people hypnotize themselves more easily than others. If you can follow directions and are willing to be hypnotized, you CAN be hypnotized. Even if you are at the more difficult end of the spectrum, you can still be hypnotized; the hypnotist just has to work a little more at getting you hypnotized. (I monitor the external signs of hypnosis in my clients to determine when they go into a trance and continue to use appropriate hypnosis-inducing language until they do so.)

Fact: Hypnosis is a learned skill. You can learn to hypnotize yourself easily and accomplish many of the changes that you desire. I teach my clients how to use self-hypnosis to achieve their goals.

Myth #8:

I have never been hypnotized before.

Basis: You have never seen a hypnotist or hypnotherapist.

Fact: Every person naturally enters a state of hypnosis at least twice every day: just before falling asleep at night, and upon awaking every morning before getting out of bed. Formal hypnosis simply duplicates the relaxed, partly drowsy, highly-suggestible state of those two times.

Fact: Most people easily enter a state of *environment hypnosis* while at the movies, watching TV, driving on the highway, or reading a good book.

Fact: You were probably hypnotized by your parents for your first few years of childhood (until you figured out how to hypnotize them!)

Fact: If you are an athlete, you experience hypnosis as *getting into the zone.*

Fact: If you have ever been in love, you experienced the ultimate hypnotic state!

Myth #9:

After hypnosis, I will have no memory of the session and won't know what happened.

Basis: You don't remember things from when you are asleep or unconscious.

Fact: Hypnosis is not an unconscious state or sleep. In fact, most people report having a heightened sense of awareness, concentration, and focus. You will have a conversation with me as your hypnotist during the session. I will instruct you to remember everything. You will get some reminders of the session to take home with you as reinforcements afterward.

Myth #10:
Hypnosis is not effective or takes a lot of expensive sessions.

Basis: Many types of therapy take a lot of sessions, so hypnosis must take many sessions too.

Fact: Hypnosis is very effective. Many hospitals use some form of hypnosis to prepare patients for surgery and assist their rapid recovery. Hypnosis is *THE* most effective method of releasing the tobacco habit.

Fact: Some issues can be solved with a single hypnosis session reinforced by personal self-hypnosis. More deeply entrenched issues take a few sessions.

Fact: Here is the hypnosis effectiveness statistics, results of a comparative study published in American Health Magazine:

- *Psychoanalysis therapy* has, on average, 38% recovery after 600 sessions.
- *Behavior therapy* has, on average, 72% recovery after 22 sessions.
- *Hypnotherapy* has, on average, 93% recovery after 6 sessions.

> *(Statistics gathered by Dr. Alfred Barrios, PhD and documented at: www.stresscards.com/hypnotherapy_reappraisal.php)*

Myth #11:
I will do embarrassing things, such as imitate a dog, chicken, or duck.

Basis: Observing entertainment hypnosis where the volunteers do these things when instructed by the hypnotist.

Fact: This myth results from confusion of therapeutic clinical hypnosis with entertainment hypnosis (stage hypnosis). Stage hypnosis follows a fixed format for entertainment.

Here is how stage hypnosis works:

1. A stage hypnotist is hired to entertain a group.

2. The hypnotist asks for volunteers who want to be hypnotized.

3. Volunteers from the group come up on stage. Most of them are just curious.

4. By volunteering, they have made a tacit agreement with the hypnotist: "We are going to have fun doing whatever you say, even being silly!" They know that they can always blame anything they feel embarrassed about afterward on the hypnotist.

5. Often one or more of the volunteers has a different agenda, namely, to *bust* the hypnotist and prove that hypnosis is a fake. (I call them the *disrupters).*

6. The hypnotist's first task is to sort out these disrupters and tell them to go sit back in the audience. (If you have seen a stage show, you may remember seeing the hypnotist send someone off the stage).

7. The hypnotist then hypnotizes the volunteers.

8. The hypnotist gives them some silly things to do and they do them (to varying degrees).

9. Those hypnotized have a choice to accept or reject the suggestions to act like a chicken or dog, and many accept them! (Perhaps they will deny their choice later because of embarrassment or some other reason).

10. The hypnotist may tell people to be "rigid as a piece of steel" and then support them horizontally by only head and heels. (This demonstrates the extreme power of your subconscious mind over your body because staying stiff horizontally is something you cannot do consciously!)

11. The hypnotist may give a temporary post-hypnotic suggestion, such as "You will forget the number 3."

12. The hypnotist brings the individual out of trance and has them count the fingers on their hand. Invariably they will say: "1, 2, 4, 5, 6," and be totally confused about how they got 6 fingers on that hand,

13. Alternatively, the hypnotist may instruct a person to "Jump up and cheer whenever I say *blue.*"

14. During a conversation, when the hypnotist casually says *blue* the person involuntarily jumps up and cheers but doesn't really understand why he did it. Some inner impulse just caused him to do it.

15. Everybody laughs and has fun, and the awesome power behind hypnosis is revealed as available for therapeutic or performance use.

Fact: Entertainment is never part of therapeutic hypnosis, which is a serious process of self-improvement. Understanding aspects of how entertainment hypnosis works is useful because the powerful aspects of hypnosis that are used in stage hypnosis are equally available for therapeutic and performance hypnosis:

Fact: You accept suggestions more easily when hypnotized.

Fact: Your subconscious has powerful control over your body and can demonstrate that control in hypnosis. (It has that same control at all times. That is why medical hypnosis is so powerful. Giving your subconscious instructions to repair and restore your body will accelerate healing.)

Fact: Post-hypnotic suggestions work automatically without thought because they come from the subconscious.

Conclusion: HYPNOSIS MYTHS BUSTED!

Now that you know better, utilize the safe power of hypnosis to get the life that you want. You can banish discomfort, repair your body, eliminate illness, add skills, drop useless habits and increase your performance and joy. See the products page at the back of the book or go to *store.DuncanTooley.com* for more information.

Still have questions about hypnosis?

Call me at *310-832-0830* or send an email to me at: *Duncan @ DuncanTooley.com*

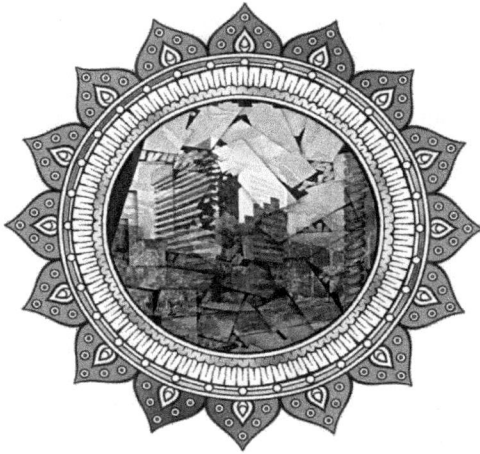

REFERENCES

Abaci, Peter. *Take Charge of Your Chronic Pain: The Latest Research, Cutting-Edge Tools, and Alternative Treatments for Feeling Better.* Guilford, CT.: GPP Life, 2010. Print.

Alidina, Shamash, and Steven D. Hickman. *Mindfulness for Dummies.* Chichester, West Sussex, Eng.: John Wiley & Sons, 2010. Print.

Allen, Claudia Kay. *The Prevention Pain-Relief System: A Total Program for Relieving Any Pain in Your Body.* Emmaus, PA: Rodale; 1992. Print.

Barsky, Arthur J., and Emily Deans. *Stop Being Your Symptoms and Start Being Yourself: The 6-week Mind-Body Program to Ease Your Chronic Symptoms.* New York, NY: Collins, 2006. Print.

Benor, Daniel J. *Seven Minutes to Natural Pain Release: WHEE for Tapping Your Pain Away, the Revolutionary New Self-healing Method.* Santa Rosa, CA: Energy Psychology, 2008. Print.

Bourke, Joanna. *The Story of Pain: From Prayer to Painkillers.* New York, NY: Oxford UP, 2014. Print.

Brady, Scott, and William Proctor. *Pain-Free for Life: The 6-Week Cure for Chronic Pain -- Without Surgery or Drugs.* New York, NY: Center Street, 2006. Print.

Brand, Paul W., and Philip Yancey. *Pain: The Gift Nobody Wants.* New York, NY: HarperCollins, 1993. Print.

Brittain, Amy. *American Cancer Society's Guide to Pain Control: Understanding and Managing Cancer Pain.* Rev. ed. Atlanta, GA.: American Cancer Society, 2004. Print.

Brown, Mark. *Conquer Back and Neck Pain - Walk It Off! A Spine Doctor's Proven Solutions for Finding Relief Without Pills or Surgery.* North Branch, MN: Sunrise River, 2008. Print.

Burch, Vidyamala. *You Are Not Your Pain: Using Mindfulness to Relieve Pain, Reduce Stress, and Restore Well-Being---an Eight-week Program.* New York, NY: Flatiron Books, 2013.Print.

Carey, Anthony. *The Pain-Free Program: A Proven Method to Relieve Back, Neck, Shoulder, and Joint Pain.* Hoboken, NJ: J. Wiley, 2005. Print.

Caudill, Margaret. *Managing Pain before It Manages You.* Rev. ed. New York: Guilford, 2002. Print.

Chillot, Rick, and Wayne Michaud. *The Anti-Pain Plan: 467 No-Nonsense Ways to Avoid Arthritis, Heal a Headache, Beat a Backache, Trounce Carpal Tunnel, Relieve Sore Joints, and More!* Wixom, MI: American Master Products/Jerry Baker, 2003. Print.

Cook, Allan R. *Pain Sourcebook.* Detroit, MI: Omnigraphics, 1998. Print.

Dyer, Wayne W., and Saje Dyer. *Good-Bye, Bumps!: Talking to What's Bugging You.* Carlsbad, CA: Hay House, 2014. Print.

Foreman, Judy. *A Nation in Pain: Healing Our Nation's Biggest Health Problem.* New York, NY: Oxford UP, 2015.Print.

Hicks, Michael D. *The Cleveland Clinic Guide to Pain Management.* New York, NY: Kaplan Pub., 2010. Print.

Hitzmann, Sue. *The Melt Method: A Breakthrough Self-Treatment System to Eliminate Chronic Pain, Erase the Signs of Aging, and Feel Fantastic in Just 10 Minutes a Day!* New York, NY: HarperOne, 2013. Print.

Kabat-Zinn, Jon, and Richard Davidson, eds. *The Mind's Own Physician: A Scientific Dialogue with the Dalai Lama on the Healing Power of Meditation.* Oakland, CA: New Harbinger Publications, 2012. Print.

REFERENCES

Kamen, Paula. *All in My Head: An Epic Quest to Cure an Unrelenting, Totally Unreasonable, and Only Slightly Enlightening Headache.* Cambridge, MA: Da Capo Lifelong, 2005. Print.

Kaplan, Gary, and Donna Beecher. *Total Recovery: Solving the Mystery of Chronic Pain and Depression : How We Get Sick, Why We Stay Sick, How We Can Recover.* New York, NY: Rodale, 2014. Print.

Kassan, S. S., and Charles J. Vierck. *Chronic Pain for Dummies.* Hoboken, NJ: Wiley Pub., 2008. Print.

Khalsa, Dharma Singh, and Cameron Stauth. *The Pain Cure: The Proven Medical Program That Helps End Your Chronic Pain.* New York, NY: Warner, 1999. Print.

Lehndorff, Peter G., and Brian Tarcy. *60 Second Chronic Pain Relief: The Quickest Way to Soften the Throb, Cool the Burn, Ease the Ache.* Far Hills, NJ: New Horizon, 1997. Print.

Lenarz, Michael, and Victoria George. *The Chiropractic Way: How Chiropractic Care Can Stop Your Pain and Help You Regain Your Health without Drugs or Surgery.* Bantam Trade Pbk. ed. New York, NY: Bantam, 2003. Print.

Levine, Peter A., and Maggie Phillips. *Freedom from Pain: Discover Your Body's Power to Overcome Physical Pain.* Boulder, CO: Sounds True, 2012. Print.

Marcus, Norman J., and Jean S. Arbeiter. *Freedom from Chronic Pain: The Breakthrough Method of Pain Relief, Based on the New York Pain Treatment Program at Lenox Hill Hospital.* New York, NY: Simon & Schuster, 1994. Print.

McCall, Timothy B. *Yoga as Medicine: The Yogic Prescription for Health & Healing: A Yoga Journal Book.* New York, NY: Bantam, 2007. Print.

McGonigal, Kelly. *Yoga for Pain Relief: Simple Practices to Calm Your Mind & Heal Your Chronic Pain.* Oakland, CA: New Harbinger Publications, 2009. Print.

Nielsen, Patricia D. *Living With It Daily: Meditations for People with Chronic Pain.* New York, NY: Dell Pub., 1994. Print.

Ortner, Nick. *The Tapping Solution for Pain Relief: A Step-by-Step Guide to Reducing and Eliminating Chronic Pain.* Carlsbad, CA: HayHouse, 2015. Print.

Oxenhandler, Harry S. *The Humpty Dumpty Syndrome: Lift Yourself from Back Pain without Drugs or Surgery.* Corvallis, OR: Master's Plan Pub. L.L.C., 2003. Print.

Patt, Richard B., and Susan S. Lang. *The Complete Guide to Relieving Cancer Pain and Suffering.* Rev. and Expanded ed. Oxford: Oxford UP, 2004. Print.

Prudden, Bonnie. *Pain Erasure: The Bonnie Prudden Way*. New York, NY: M. Evans, 1980. Print.

Richard, Diana. *Healthy Joints for Life : An Orthopedic Surgeon's Proven Plan to Reduce Pain and Inflammation, Avoid Surgery and Get Moving Again*. Ontario, Canada: Harlequin, 1960. Print.

Richeimer, Steven, and Kathy Steligo. *Confronting Chronic Pain: A Pain Doctor's Guide to Relief*. Baltimore, MD: Johns Hopkins UP, 2014. Print.

St. Cecile C. M., and Christine Buttinger. *Relieving Pelvic Pain during and after Pregnancy: How Women Can Heal Chronic Pelvic Instability*. Alameda, CA: Hunter House, 2007. Print.

Saper, Joel R., and Kenneth R. Magee. *Freedom from Headaches: A Personal Guide for Understanding and Treating Headache, Face, and Neck Pain*. New York, NY: Simon and Schuster, 1978. Print.

Sarno, John E. *Healing Back Pain: The Mind-Body Connection*. New York, NY: Warner, 1991. Print.

Schatz, Mary Pullig. *Back Care Basics: A Doctor's Gentle Yoga Program for Back and Neck Pain Relief*. Berkeley, CA: Rodmell, 1992. Print.

Silver, J. K. *Chronic Pain and the Family: A New Guide*. Cambridge, MA: Harvard UP, 2004. Print.

Silverman, Gerald M. *Your Miraculous Back: A Step-by-Step Guide to Relieving Neck & Back Pain*. Oakland, CA: New Harbinger Publications, 2006. Print.

Skrobisch, Al. *Pain Relief for Life*. Franklin Lakes, NJ: New Page, 2003. Print.

Starlanyl, Devin, and Mary Ellen Copeland. *Fibromyalgia & Chronic Myofascial Pain Syndrome: A Survival Manual*. Oakland, CA: New Harbinger Publications, 1996. Print.

Tick, Heather. *Holistic Pain Relief: Dr. Tick's Breakthrough Strategies to Manage and Eliminate Pain*. Novato, CA: New World Library. Print.

Valdez, Joseph, and Miguel Pappolla. *Healing Back and Joint Injuries: A Proven Approach to Ending Chronic Pain and Avoiding Unnecessary Surgery*. Austin, TX.: Greenleaf Book Group, 2009. Print.

Vlachonis, Vicky, and Mariska Van Aalst. *The Body Doesn't Lie: A 3-step Program to End Chronic Pain and Become Positively Radiant*. New York: Harper Collins, 2014. Print.

STUDY REFERENCES

Study 1: "Preoperative Instruction for Decreased Bleeding During Spine Surgery," *Anesthesiology* 1986; 65:A245.

Study 2: Kathleen Haralson, *Professional's Guide to Exercise and Medical Conditions*, IDEA Health & *Fitness, 2000*, ISBN=188778117X

Study 3: "The Truth About the Truth: a meta-analytic review of the Truth Effect," *Personality and Social Psychology Review* in May 2010 (14(2):238-57).

Study 4: "A Randomized Clinical Trial of a Brief Hypnosis Intervention to Control Side Effects in Breast Surgery Patients," *Journal of the National Cancer Institute,* 2007 Sep 99(17):1304-12.

Study 5: *usatoday30.usatoday.com/news/health/2005-05-09-prayer-pain_x.htm*

Study 6: "Rapid Changes in Histone Deacetylases and Inflammatory Gene Expression in Expert Meditators," *Psychoneuroendocrinology.* 2014 Feb;40: 96–107.

Study 7: Timothy McCall, MD, *Yoga As Medicine,* (See entry for book in complete reference list).

Study 8: "Yoga for Chronic Neck Pain: A Pilot Randomized Controlled Clinical Trial," *Journal of Pain*, 2012 Nov;13(11):1122-30.

Study 9: "Beautiful Art Eases Pain," *University World News,* Oct 5, 2008; Issue No:47, www.universityworldnews.com/article.php?story=20081002145858911

Study 10: "A Dose of Music for Pain Relief," *Society for Neuroscience*, Jan 2013, reported by BrainFacts.org www.brainfacts.org/sensing-thinking-behaving/senses-and-perception/articles/2013/a-dose-of-music-for-pain-relief/

Study 11: Dr. Kevin Berry, TMJ Therapy & Sleep Center of Colorado; www.tmjtherapyandsleepcenter.com/chronic-pain-relief-for-a-song/

Study 12: "A Randomized Trial of Tai Chi for Fibromyalgia," *New England Journal of Medicine,* 2010 Aug 19; 363(8):743-54.

Study 13: "Hypnosis in Contemporary Medicine, "Mayo *Clinic Proceedings* 2005; 80:511-524.

Study 14: "Intensive Therapy: Utilizing Hypnosis in the Treatment of Substance Abuse Disorders," Potter, Greg, *American Journal of Clinical Hypnosis*, Jul 2004.

Study 15: "A Comparative Study of Hypnotherapy and Psychotherapy in the Treatment of Methadone Addicts," *American Journal of Clinical Hypnosis*, 1984; 26(4): 273-9.

Study16: "Hypnosis as an Adjunct to Cognitive-Behavioral Psychotherapy for Obesity: A Meta-Analytic Reappraisal," *Journal Consult Clinical Psychol.* 1996; 64(3):513-516.

Study 17: "How One in Five Give Up Smoking," *Journal of Applied Psychology*, October 1992.

Study 18: "Effect of Guided Imagery on Length of Stay, Pain and Anxiety in Cardiac Surgery Patients," *Journal of Cardiovascular Management* 10;2:22-8 1999

Study 19: "A Randomized Clinical Trial of a Brief Hypnosis Intervention to Control Side Effects in Breast Surgery Patients," *Journal of the National Cancer Institute*, 2007 Sep; 99(17):1304-12.

Study 20: "fMRI Used to Investigate Brain Activity Under Hypnosis for Pain Suppression," *Regional Anesthesia and Pain Medicine,* Nov-Dec 2004.

Study 21: "Controlled Trial of Hypnotherapy in the Treatment of Refractory Fibromyalgia," Netherlands, *Journal of Rheumatology 1991, vol. 18, no1, pp. 72-75*

Study 22: "Hypnosis in Dermatology," *Dermatol.* 2000 Mar;136(3):393-9

Study 23: "The Treatment of Irritable Bowel Syndrome with Hypnotherapy," *Appl Psychophysiol Biofeedback.* 1998 Dec;23(4):219-32

Study 24: "Effect of Preoperative Suggestion on Postoperative Gastro-intestinal Motility," *West J Med* 1993 158;5:488-92

Study 25: "Hypnosis Slows Impacts of Dementia and Improves Quality of Life," (www.liv.ac.uk/researchintelligence/issue36/hypnosis.htm), University of Liverpool Research Intelligence.

Study 26: "Can Medical Hypnosis Accelerate Post-Surgical Wound Healing? Results of a Clinical Trial," *Am J Clin Hypn.* 2003 Apr;45(4):333-51.

Study 27: "Using Hypnosis to Accelerate the Healing of Bone Fractures: A Randomized Controlled Pilot Study," *Alter Ther Health Med.* 1999 Mar; 5(2):67-75

Study 28: "The Use of Hypnosis in the Treatment of Burn Patients," *International Handbook of Clinical Hypnosis,* Online ISBN: 9780470846407; DOI=10.1002/ 0470846402.ch19

Study 29: "Hypnotherapy for Incontinence Caused by the Unstable Detrusor." *Br Med J (Clin Res Ed).* 1982 June 19; 284(6332): 1831–1834.

STUDY REFERENCES

Study 30: "Efficacy of Testosterone, Trazodone and Hypnotic Suggestion in the Treatment of Non-Organic Male Sexual Dysfunction," Yüzüncü Yil University, Van, Turkey. *Br J Urol.* 1996 Feb;77(2):256-60.

Study 31: "Medical Hypnosis: An Underutilized Treatment Approach," *Permanente Journal,* Fall 2001/Vol. 5, No. 4.

Study 32: "Hypnosis with Conscious Sedation Instead of General Anesthesia? Applications in Cervical Endocrine Surgery," University of Liege, Belgium, *Acta Chir Belg.* 1999 Aug;99(4):151-8.

Study 33: "Cognitive Restructuring: A Technique for the Relief of Chronic Tinnitus," *Australian Journal of Clinical and Experimental Hypnosis,* 10 (1), 27-33.

Study 34: "An Alternative Method of Treating Tinnitus: Relaxation-Hypnotherapy Primarily through the Home Use of a Recorded Audio Cassette," *International Journal of Clinical and Experimental Hypnosis,* 31 (2), 90-97.

Study 35: "Successful Aging through Digital Games: Socioemotional Differences between Older Adult Gamers and Non-gamers," *Computers in human Behavior,* 2013 July; (29 (4):1302–6.

Study 36: "Mind-Body Hypnotic Imagery in the Treatment of Auto-Immune Disorders," Moshe S. Torem, *American Journal of Clinical Hypnosis,* 50:2, 157-170, DOI:10.1080/00029157.2007.10401612

Study 37: "Hypnosis: An Alternate Approach to Insomnia," Donald C. Paterson, PMCID: PMC2306547, *Can Fam Physician.* 1982 Apr; 28: 768–770.

Study 38: "Hypnosis for Nausea and Vomiting in Cancer Chemotherapy: a Systematic Review of the Research Evidence," Richardson J, *Eur J Cancer Care (Engl).* 2007 Sep;16(5):402-12

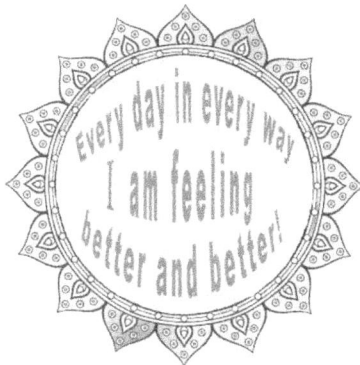

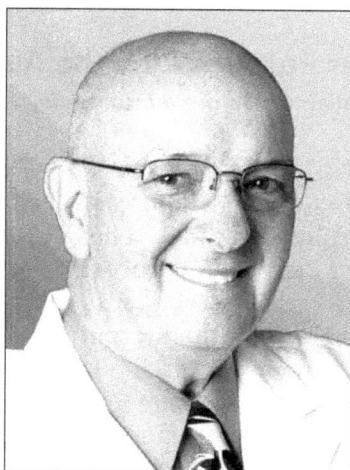

ABOUT THE AUTHOR

Duncan Tooley is a mind trainer, medical hypnotherapist, artist, author, speaker, and life coach. He teaches others to change their thinking, beliefs, and habits. This results in pain-free, lower-weight, less-stressed clients feeling themselves more in control of their health and emotions.

As a Catholic religious bother, Duncan taught high school science for 7 years before beginning his 35-year secular career in corporate information technology interrupted by disabling neuropathy. After years of ineffective medical treatment, he discovered hypnosis and used it to clear his illness. This transformation, and its accompanying spiritual awakening, inspired his career change to become a mind trainer, medical hypnotist, and coach specializing in weight reduction and pain relief. (See his story in the Preface).

Duncan is a lifelong artist, creator of a unique hypnotic weight loss program, Toastmasters International speaker, presenter to cancer support organizations, and Certified Hypnosis Instructor (CHI) for the International Hypnosis Federation.

Other Resources by the Author
available at: *store.duncantooley.com*

Healthy & Feeling Great
- *Medical Benefits of Hypnosis* – free report
- *Feel Great* hypnotic pain relief & wellness meditation
- *60-second Pain Relief* process
- *Pain Gone* word search puzzle
- *More Fun Exercise* meditation
- *Anti-Anxious* word search puzzles
- *Self-Hypnosis to Accelerate Healing* multimedia meditation
- *Knockout Stress* multimedia experience
- *Restful Sleep Expels Insomnia* meditation

Positivity-Creativity-Art-Fun
- *Tooley's Law* (of Attraction) – free audio
- *Principles of Tooley's Law* (of Attraction)
- *Fun Creative Art* word search puzzle
- *Creative Mandala Experience* multimedia meditation
- *Positive Aspects* word search puzzles
- *Ace My Exam or Final Grade* meditation experience
- *Increase Anything* meditation experience

Nutrition & Weight
- *Think Myself SLIM® Weight Loss System* – free sample
- *Turn Your Fat Burner UP* hypnotic meditation
- *Healthy Eating* word search puzzle
- *End My French Fry Craving* multimedia
- *Turn OFF ANY Craving* multimedia meditation
- *Tapping Away Overeating* acupressure process

Resource information at **store.*duncantooley.com***

Email Contact: *duncan@duncantooley.com*
Or call **310-832-0830**
Also see artworks by the author at: ***www.TooleyArtStudio.com,***
and more pain-related information at: ***www.painhypnotist.com***

www.ingramcontent.com/pod-product-compliance
Lightning Source LLC
Chambersburg PA
CBHW071544200326
41519CB00021BB/6611